"Packed with useful tools, ines, this well-written book is a gold mine for the tep-by-step, it will help you to develop all the skill challenges of this specialized field. If you do acceptance and commitment (ACT), and you work with psychotic clients, then you can't afford to go without this book!"

—**Russ Harris**, author of *The Happiness Trap* and *ACT Made Simple*

"*ACT for Psychosis Recovery* is a fantastic resource for anyone wishing to offer ACT groups for people experiencing psychosis, or for their caregivers. It is written by leading experts in the field, and includes a thorough overview of theory and evidence. The inclusion of a chapter on peer-support co-facilitation is welcome and is in keeping with the values base of the approach. The group manual itself is very comprehensive, covering each session in detail and including a number of prompt sheets. These will help practitioners put the manual into practice with confidence."

—**Clara Strauss, DPhil, DClinPsych**, consultant clinical psychologist and clinical research fellow and research lead at Sussex Mindfulness Centre, University of Sussex, and Sussex Partnership NHS Foundation Trust

"This book is an absolute must for any mental health clinician who wants to provide state-of-the-art, evidence-based care to clients suffering from psychotic experiences, whether it be on the inpatient ward, or in an outpatient community setting.… The manual is supported by numerous worksheets, detailed instructions for conducting core ACT metaphors in session, and helpful hints for addressing common issues. The authors demonstrate an unrivaled depth of knowledge of, and compassion for, those whose lives are affected by psychosis. That alone would make this book a key addition to any mental health clinician's library!"

—**Kirk Strosahl PhD**, cofounder of ACT, and coauthor of *The Mindfulness and Acceptance Workbook for Depression*

"As a direct result of my participation in ACT, and practicing the essential taught tools, ACT for psychosis recovery disrupted my revolving door, long sessions in locked psychiatric hospitals, and led to my learning how to productively identify constructive approaches and manage challenges to ensure my enjoyment daily, of a quality of life with my mental health diagnoses, that had been denied to me before this therapy. Prior to ACT, my psychosis was indeed so pronounced, aggressive, and bleak, that I also spent time in prison. ACT for psychosis recovery was my final attempt at therapy."

—**Yvonne Patricia Stewart-Williams**, artist, and author of *Still On The Cusp Of Madness*

"Compiled by experts in the field, this is a comprehensive and invaluable resource for supporting recovery in the context of psychosis. Written in an engaging and accessible way, the importance of close collaboration with experienced experts is highlighted throughout. The authors are to be commended for developing an approach that richly recognizes the common humanity shared by those who have experienced psychosis, and those who are committed to helping."

—**Ross G. White, PhD, DClinPsy**, associate professor of clinical psychology at the University of Liverpool

"As evidence of the benefits of ACT for psychosis are piling up, there is a need for a clear and practical manual on how to implement ACT for psychosis in the clinical workplace. This book is offering exactly that, an extensive and detailed manual of a four-session ACT group intervention for people suffering from psychosis at different stages of illness, as well as their caregivers. With additional information on training, supervision, and inclusion of peer-support co-facilitators, this book is a must-read for all clinicians interested in third-wave psychotherapies for people with psychosis."

—**Inez Myin-Germeys**, professor of psychiatry, and head of the Center for Contextual Psychiatry at KU Leuven in Belgium

"ACT has enriched the family of cognitive behavioral therapies immeasurably. This book distills over ten years of the authors' work developing ACT for and with people struggling with psychosis. *ACT for Psychosis Recovery* provides detailed guidance on how to run groups for people with psychosis, and their caregivers. In the spirit of generosity associated with ACT, the book includes all the worksheets, metaphors, and measures needed to run these groups in clinical practice."

—**Katherine Newman-Taylor**, consultant clinical psychologist at Southern Health NHS Foundation Trust, and associate professor at the University of Southampton

"*ACT for Psychosis Recovery* is a unique resource for practitioners from any background. Developed by expert clinicians who are also leading researchers, the manual shows how to engage participants in simple and powerful group exercises that foster hope and enable action today toward living a more satisfying life. The use of a central metaphor and straightforward language accommodates all abilities, and innovations in peer facilitation and caregiver groups open new directions. When implementing it in our services, the degree of change in participants surprised even our group leaders. The authors are onto something special here!"

—**John Farhall, PhD**, associate professor of clinical psychology at La Trobe University, and consultant clinical psychologist at NorthWestern Mental Health in Melbourne, Australia

ACT *for* PSYCHOSIS RECOVERY

A Practical Manual for Group-Based Interventions Using Acceptance & Commitment Therapy

Emma K. O'Donoghue, DClinPsy | Eric M.J. Morris, PhD
Joseph E. Oliver, PhD | Louise C. Johns, DPhil

CONTEXT PRESS
An Imprint of New Harbinger Publications, Inc.

Publisher's Note

This publication is designed to provide accurate and authoritative information in regard to the subject matter covered. It is sold with the understanding that the publisher is not engaged in rendering psychological, financial, legal, or other professional services. If expert assistance or counseling is needed, the services of a competent professional should be sought.

Distributed in Canada by Raincoast Books

Copyright © 2018 by Emma K. O'Donoghue, Eric M.J. Morris, Joseph E. Oliver, and Louise C. Johns
Context Press
An imprint of New Harbinger Publications, Inc.
5674 Shattuck Avenue
Oakland, CA 94609
www.newharbinger.com

Cover design by Amy Shoup

Acquired by Catharine Meyers

Edited by James Lainsbury

Indexed by James Minkin

All Rights Reserved

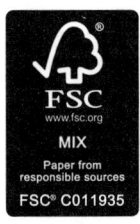 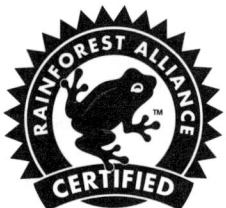

Library of Congress Cataloging-in-Publication Data on file

20 19 18

10 9 8 7 6 5 4 3 2 1   First Printing

Emma O'Donoghue
To my darling Johnny and my amazing family and friends. I love you dearly.

Joe Oliver
To my wife, Shalyn, with much love.

Eric Morris
To my parents, Nev and Bev. I am, as ever, grateful for your love and support.

Louise Johns
Per Andrea. Grazie per il tuo impegno.

Contents

Foreword ix

An Introduction to Acceptance and Commitment Therapy (ACT) for
Psychosis Recovery 1

PART 1: Pretreatment Overview

CHAPTER 1
Introduction to Acceptance and Commitment Therapy for Psychosis 7

CHAPTER 2
Adapting ACT Workshops for Caregivers of People with Psychosis 33
Written with Suzanne Jolley

CHAPTER 3
Adapting ACT Workshops for Acute Inpatient Settings 51
Written with Rumina Taylor and Georgina Bremner

CHAPTER 4
Peer-Support Cofacilitators 67
Working Alongside Clients with Lived Experience of Mental Health Issues

CHAPTER 5
Running Successful and Effective Workshops 79
Training

CHAPTER 6
Running Successful and Effective Workshops 99
Supervision and Evaluation

PART 2: Treatment Manual

Introduction to ACT for Psychosis Recovery Workshop Protocol *Written with Natasha Avery*	119
Taster Session	123
SESSION 1 Introducing Noticing, Values, and Committed Action	133
SESSION 2 Workability as an Alternative	149
SESSION 3 Acting on Values with Openness, Awareness, and Willingness	171
SESSION 4 Bringing It All Together—Open, Aware, and Active	187
Booster Session 1	201
Booster Session 2	211
Acknowledgments	221
APPENDIX A Exercise Prompt Sheets	223
A1. Reservoir Metaphor	224
A2. Mindfulness of Breath and Body Exercise	225
A3. Passengers on the Bus Metaphor	227
A4. Mindful Stretch Exercise	228
A5. Mindful Eating Exercise	230
A6. Paul's Story Transcript	232
A7. George's Story Transcript	234
A8. Pushing Against the Folder Exercise	236
A9. Acting Out the Passengers on the Bus Exercise	238
A10. Three-Minute Breathing Space Exercise	241
A11. Leaves on the Stream Exercise	242
A12. Mindful Walking Exercise	244
A13. Key Messages Cards	246
A14. Clouds in the Sky Exercise	249
A15. Client Satisfaction Questionnaire	250
A16. The ACTs of ACT Fidelity Measure	253

APPENDIX B
Session Worksheets   257
  B1. Values Worksheet   258
  B2. Passengers on the Bus Worksheet   259
  B3. Committed Action Worksheet   260
  B4. Developing Aware Skills Worksheet   261
  B5. Driving License Worksheet side 1   262
      Driving License Worksheet side 2   263

Reference List   265

Index   281

List of Figures

FIGURE 1
The ACT model of psychological flexibility, or hexaflex   12

FIGURE 2
The ACTs of ACT Fidelity Measure   105

List of Tables

TABLE 1
Central ACT processes   13

TABLE 2
The content of workshop sessions in ACT for recovery in acute
inpatient settings   61

FOREWORD

ACT for Psychosis: It Is Time

When people trot out statistics on the cost of mental health problems, they often fail to note that psychosis produces a large share of those costs. I'm not talking just about dollars and cents. People struggling with psychosis die at a far younger age; they are commonly in poverty; they are frequently victims of violent crime; and they have dramatically poorer overall physical health.

Meanwhile, the mental health establishment has been all too willing to accept that anti-psychotic medications are full and ready solutions to these problems, with psychosocial interventions playing only a minor and supportive role. As providers, family members, and recipients of care all increasingly realize: this approach is not working. All anti-psychotic medications have serious side effects that grow with time and dose. Some of these include metabolic problems and cardiovascular disease, which contribute to the health problems and lowered life expectancy I just noted. Because the use of anti-psychotic medications prematurely settled into a status of accepted community practice before the data were fully in, many of the needed studies on long-term effects were never done, leading to a serious hole in our knowledge base that we have yet to fill adequately. Existing medications do have a role in the care of psychotic patients, but it is more limited than current practice suggests. Medication as a form of intervention needs to be combined with evidence-based psychosocial methods.

In the last 15 years, there has been steady progress in the investigation of acceptance and commitment therapy (ACT) as a psychosocial method with broad applicability to the range of problems that emerge in intervention with psychosis. ACT is not a psychotherapy designed to eliminate the signs and symptoms of psychosis. The target of ACT is the empowerment of people to deal with life, including the presence of various experiences that may be challenging, such as hearing voices or having ideas of reference. ACT is focused on goals such as increasing quality of life or employment, staying out of the hospital, and reducing distress and entanglement with symptoms. Empowering people to face life's challenges, however, does not just apply to recipients of care. It applies also to family members, caregivers, and professionals.

In all of these areas, the evidence in support of ACT is growing. Take rehospitalization: there are now three completely independent studies examining the impact of very brief ACT interventions for people hospitalized with psychosis, examining its impact on rehospitalization.* All of them found significant reductions of rehospitalization over four months using survival analysis. Having a larger body of evidence available across studies now allows us to ask very simple but very important questions, like "Does ACT help keep psychotic patients out of the hospital at all?" The answer, in short, is yes. Counting all missing data as bad outcomes (the most conservative possible assumption), across these studies 46% of the treatment as usual condition were rehospitalized over 4 months, as compared to 28% in the ACT condition. That is a significant difference (Fisher's exact, $p = .037$) that represents a nearly 40% drop in the rate of rehospitalization—a number sure to get the attention of both researchers and the treatment community worldwide.

That is now happening. In 2017, scientists for the National Registry of Evidence-based Programs and Practices (NREPP) of the Substance Abuse and Mental Health Services Administration of the United States examined the ACT for psychosis studies. NREPP decided to categorize acceptance and commitment therapy as "Effective" for its impact on rehospitalization. The impact of ACT was listed as "Promising" also for psychosocial disability and overall psychiatric problems.

Supportive data is not just available for outcomes, and we now know that psychological flexibility mediates the outcome of ACT for psychosis. Longitudinal and cross-sectional studies show that the theory applies to the life impact of hallucinations and delusions as well. This all suggests that something important is going on in ACT for psychosis, and after 15 years of development work, it is time to move these methods more fully into systems of care.

This book is the first to present a comprehensive and practical approach to the full range of issues involved in the treatment of psychosis using ACT. Written by some of the leading developers in the area, it contains sections on the theory underlying ACT, how its methods fit into existing systems of care, how ACT can be done in inpatient settings using peers and cofacilitators, how

---

* The three studies that have looked at that are Bach and Hayes (2002), Gaudiano & Herbert (2006), and Tyrberg, Carlbring, & Lundgren (2017). The first two references are in the main reference list for this book. The last reference is Tyrberg, M. J., Carlbring, P. & Lundgren, T. (2017). Brief acceptance and commitment therapy for psychotic inpatients: A randomized controlled feasibility trial in Sweden. *Nordic Psychology*, 69, 110-125. Doi: 10.1080/19012276.2016.1198271

ACT applies to caregivers and providers, and how ACT can be trained and supervised. There is no other resource available that addresses such a breadth of practical topics that systems of care need to know in order to take advantage of ACT methods.

The core of the book is the group ACT for psychosis protocol itself. Well crafted, flexible, and wise, it is a protocol that can be fitted to a wide range of practice settings, and for low cost. The protocol is designed to be deployed in a handful of sessions—a restriction that anyone working in the area knows is necessary. The sessions are described in detail, but the principles and purposes are described so that modification is not difficult. Breakdowns by time help group facilitators know if they are managing their time effectively, and the protocol offers an attention to contextual details and implementation issues that can only be learned one way: by being used.

What you have here is a method that has been refined over years of implementation, presented by experts. This is not a beta-test. This is a group protocol you can use with confidence in which most of the issues you will encounter in its use have been anticipated.

We now know that evidence-based psychosocial methods are key to reducing the human costs of psychosis. The field is looking for a new way forward. This book can help you provide just that to your agency and to the lives of those you serve.

—Steven C. Hayes
University of Nevada, Reno

An Introduction to Acceptance and Commitment Therapy (ACT) for Psychosis Recovery

The experience of psychosis is almost always an incredibly disruptive event in a person's life. For the approximately 3 percent of us affected by psychosis, its impact extends to every area of life, including relationships, work, health, and overall well-being. Families and caregivers also experience this impact as they do their best to support their loved one on the path toward recovery. Heartbreakingly, recovery is not guaranteed, and even when there is success, interventions such as medications come with unpleasant side effects, and diagnostic labels are extraordinarily stigmatizing.

Psychological therapies offer hope and are often a crucial and important treatment option for individuals with psychosis. For clients in close contact with their families, treatment guidelines also recommend family interventions and caregiver support, to improve caregiver well-being and their interactions with clients. Individual psychological therapies can be complex and lengthy. In addition to training more mental health staff to deliver these therapies, briefer or group-based variants of therapy have been developed to improve both dissemination and access.

Targeting common processes that contribute to psychological well-being can increase therapy impact and access. A key component of mental well-being is psychological flexibility, which involves developing helpful responses to situations and experiences using mindful awareness and values-based choices and actions. The transdiagnostic approach of acceptance and commitment therapy (ACT) aims to increase psychological flexibility, and it has been used successfully with a wide range of mental and physical health problems in clinical and nonclinical groups.

ACT promotes social and functional recovery by shifting client focus from symptom control to connecting with personal values and participating in life more fully. In addition to enhancing values-based living, ACT may be particularly useful for symptoms of psychosis. The qualities of distressing voices and delusional beliefs can increase the likelihood that people respond either with avoidance or engagement, both of which can have high personal cost in the long term. Similarly, for caregivers the worry and demands of caring responsibilities can be overwhelming, leading to unhelpful responses to distress. The aim of ACT is to change the relationship people have with their symptoms, worries, or distress, and how they respond to them, in order to reduce the impact of these difficulties and help people focus more on valued actions.

The group context provides a powerful setting within which ACT concepts and skills can be taught and modeled. In addition, aspects of the intervention lend themselves to a group setting, such as acting out ACT metaphors, observing other people being present and willing, and making commitments in a social context. For people with psychosis, and their caregivers, group interventions also offer opportunities for normalizing and accepting psychotic experiences, gaining peer support, reducing isolation, and developing self-compassion. Along with these benefits, there is the opportunity to validate the courage and commitment participants show in expanding their lives despite the personal and wider difficulties associated with psychosis.

During the last ten years, we progressively developed an ACT for recovery group intervention for people with psychosis (G-ACTp) and for their caregivers. This process has been gradual and iterative, as we've sought to create a successful, engaging, and effective group program for both individuals affected by distressing psychosis and caregivers and family members walking alongside them in the journey to recovery. We are incredibly grateful for all the feedback, suggestions, and ideas we've received over the course of this enormous project. Given the difficulties some people have accessing individual and family therapies, and the fact that there are benefits of group approaches, we believe that G-ACTp offers promise in expanding the choice and availability of high-quality psychological therapies, which can positively impact people on the pathway to recovery.

Structure of the Book

This book details the various aspects of our ACT for recovery group intervention, describing adaptations we have made and providing the manualized session content. Chapter 1 introduces ACT and its application to psychosis and outlines the development of the group intervention. Chapters 2 and 3 describe adaptations to the protocol for use with caregivers and acute inpatients, respectively. Chapter 4 details the approach of training and supervising peer-support cofacilitators, including the practical considerations and the perspectives of peer-support facilitators who have been involved. Chapter 5 discusses skills and tips for running successful workshops, both in relation to your own practice and in training others to facilitate these workshops. Chapter 6 highlights the importance of ongoing supervision and using ratings to ensure adherence to the model, and in it we consider how to measure outcomes and processes of change in the workshops. Part 2 describes the protocol for running ACT for recovery group intervention workshops; we outline each session, including scripts for exercises and tips about how to present material and foster discussion. We also provide downloadable resources at the website for this book, http://www.actforpsychosis.com, as well as advice about how to produce your own resources that better fit your service setting.

We hope you find that the book and additional resources enrich your clinical practice as you walk together with your clients on the journey to recovery!

PART 1

Pretreatment Overview

CHAPTER 1

Introduction to Acceptance and Commitment Therapy for Psychosis

In this chapter we give a brief overview of psychosis and psychological treatment approaches. We introduce acceptance and commitment therapy (ACT) and its application to psychosis, and then outline the development of our ACT for recovery group intervention.

Given that antipsychotic medication is not well tolerated, is only partially effective, and can have harmful side effects (Furukawa et al., 2015; Lieberman et al., 2005), psychological therapies offer a vital treatment option for clients. International clinical guidelines recommend that people with psychosis are offered individual cognitive behavioral therapy (CBT; Gaebel, Riesbeck, & Wobrock, 2011), but access remains limited in front-line services, mainly due to a lack of trained therapists. To help meet demand, group-based CBT interventions have been evaluated, as these can be offered to more clients at a time and can also be manualized and taught within services to increase the scope of their delivery.

ACT is a contextual cognitive behavioral intervention that lends itself to brief group therapy and to the diverse presentations of psychosis. Rather than targeting particular appraisals, as in traditional CBT, the ACT approach is not symptom specific. It emphasizes the person's relationship with symptoms and encourages values-based living (Hayes, 2004). ACT concepts and skills can be taught and modeled within a group format, plus this approach can appeal to clients who are unable or reluctant to engage with lengthy individual treatments. In addition to these aspects of ACT, the development of our workshops was also informed by our local context and the clients accessing the service, many of whom had histories of marginalization, low educational achievement, and a distrust of authority figures. We wanted to offer a brief group intervention that would be engaging, nonthreatening, and usable by clients in their daily lives.

Psychosis

Psychosis is a broad concept that is something of an umbrella term for lots of different experiences. Clinicians use the term to refer to the positive symptoms of psychotic disorders: unusual beliefs (delusions), anomalous experiences (hallucinations and other perceptual changes), and disturbances of thought and language. Individuals experiencing psychosis may say that people are trying to harm them in some way, or that they are being controlled by an external agent, and they may hear voices insulting them or commanding them to do things against their will. Their thoughts may be jumbled or experienced as inserted into, or stolen from, their mind, and thought disturbances can manifest as tangential or circumstantial speech. Although psychotic experiences are hallmark symptoms of schizophrenia, they also occur with other problems, such as mood and personality disorders, and they are reported by people who don't have a psychiatric diagnosis (Kelleher & DeVylder, 2017; McGrath et al., 2015). People diagnosed with a psychotic disorder, particularly schizophrenia, are also likely to experience negative symptoms, such as lack of motivation and reduced emotional expression, plus cognitive problems of poor memory and concentration. It's worth keeping in mind that all these symptoms can be accompanied—and often preceded—by more common emotional difficulties, such as anxiety and depression (Birchwood, 2003). It is also worth noting that psychotic experiences are not always experienced as unwanted or distressing, and they do not necessarily result in a need for care (Brett, Peters, & McGuire, 2015; Linscott & van Os, 2013).

Outcomes Following Psychosis

Diagnosable psychotic disorders affect 3 percent of the population. So, in a group of 100,000, that works out to be 3,000 people. Psychosis is considered a "severe mental illness," and it tends to reduce quality of life, social inclusion, and employment opportunities for both service users and family members (Schizophrenia Commission, 2012). It has societal costs as well, including expensive crisis care and clients and caregivers not being able to work to their full potential (Knapp et al., 2014). Psychosis is also associated with an increased risk of physical health problems and early mortality (Hjorthøj, Stürup, McGrath, & Nordentoft, 2017), as well as increased risk of suicide (Nordentoft, Madsen, & Fedyszyn, 2015).

Although individuals who develop psychosis can have a favorable prognosis, recovery rates are variable. Also, even if an individual's psychotic symptoms improve, the person may not achieve a full social and functional recovery.

In the AESOP–10 follow-up study of 557 individuals who experienced a first episode of psychosis in the United Kingdom (Morgan et al., 2014), clinical outcomes were better than social outcomes: almost half of the people in the study didn't have any psychotic symptoms for at least two years, whereas the majority experienced social exclusion (for example, being unemployed or not being in a relationship). In a systematic review of recovery in nonaffective psychoses, Jääskeläinen and colleagues (2013) found that only one in seven individuals met their criteria for both clinical and social recovery. Unfortunately, despite more treatment options in recent decades, such as newer medications and psychological therapies, the proportion of those who recover fully has not improved over time.

Definitions of recovery include "living a satisfying, hopeful and contributing life even with limitations caused by the illness" (Anthony, 1993, p. 527), and factors important in recovery include having a sense of purpose and direction (Deegan, 1988) and developing valued social roles (Slade, 2009). These factors are included in the CHIME framework for personal recovery in mental health (Leamy, Bird, Le Boutillier, Williams, & Slade, 2011), which we return to later in the chapter. CHIME is a handy acronym for:

connectedness (connecting with others),

hope (finding and maintaining hope and optimism),

identity (reestablishing a positive identity),

meaning (finding meaning in life), and

empowerment (taking responsibility for one's life, or self-management).

There are lots of reasons why recovery can be a significant challenge for many people with psychosis. Along with unusual experiences, negative symptoms, and cognitive problems, people can struggle with changes in emotional well-being and their sense of identity. In addition, due to the stigma of severe mental illness, people can feel shame and alienation from their communities.

Psychological Interventions for Psychosis

Psychological interventions, for both clients and caregivers, are now an accepted part of routine care and are recommended by international health care guidelines (Dixon et al., 2010; Gaebel et al., 2011; National Institute for Health and Care Excellence, 2014). Cognitive behavioral therapy for psychosis

(CBTp) is an adaptation of CBT for emotional disorders, tailored to the specific difficulties of people with psychosis. Therapy involves working toward personal recovery goals, and its focus includes positive psychotic symptoms, emotional problems, and negative symptoms. Overall, the evidence shows that it is relatively effective, with small to medium treatment effects (Jauhar et al., 2014; National Institute for Health and Care Excellence, 2014; van der Gaag, Valmaggia, & Smit, 2014). Individual family interventions focus on the areas of understanding psychosis, problem solving, emotional warmth, and communication among family members; improving caregiver well-being and interactions with service users; and reducing relapse and readmission rates (National Institute for Health and Care Excellence, 2014).

Despite the recommendations, the effective implementation of psychological interventions in psychosis services remains limited (Schizophrenia Commission, 2012). These therapies can be complex and lengthy, and their delivery in routine service has been restricted by low numbers of therapists, limited access to adequate training and supervision, and a lack of protected time for staff to deliver the interventions (Ince, Haddock, & Tai, 2015). The high cost of training and supervising psychological therapists in sufficient numbers to meet demand has led researchers and clinicians to evaluate briefer or group-based variants of CBTp, which have the potential to improve both its dissemination and accessibility. However, the evidence base for these treatments remains limited, and they have had a modular focus targeting particular symptoms or problems rather than psychosis more broadly (Freeman et al., 2015; Waller, Freeman, Jolley, Dunn, & Garety, 2011).

Although targeted interventions are effective, when they are applied one after another they can add up to lengthy therapies, restricting their usefulness in busy services with limited numbers of staff trained to deliver these interventions. In addition, people with psychosis often have other problems, such as health concerns, trauma, and emotional difficulties. Another approach to increasing therapy impact and access is to target common processes that contribute to psychological well-being, regardless of diagnosis. A core component of mental well-being is psychological flexibility (Kashdan & Rottenberg, 2010), which involves developing helpful responses to situations and experiences by using acceptance, mindful awareness, choice, and values-based actions. The transdiagnostic approach of ACT aims to increase psychological flexibility, and this approach has been applied successfully to a wide range of mental and physical health problems for which flexibility processes are limited or reduced.

Acceptance and Commitment Therapy (ACT)

Acceptance and commitment therapy (ACT) belongs to a group of third-wave, or contextual cognitive behavioral therapeutic, approaches that emphasizes altering the way people relate to their thinking and feeling, rather than directly trying to change the form or frequency of these internal experiences (Hayes, 2004). The ACT model is underpinned by a behavioral analytic account of language called relational frame theory (RFT; Blackledge, Ciarrochi, & Deane, 2009), and therapy aims to reduce the impact of thoughts and language in order to increase the amount of choice one has with regard to following a valued life path.

ACT aims to increase psychological flexibility by helping people develop mindfulness and noticing skills, engage in values-based actions, and reduce the processes of experiential avoidance and cognitive fusion that exacerbate negative emotional states and limit functioning (Hayes, Luoma, Bond, Masuda, & Lillis, 2006; Hayes, Strosahl, & Wilson 2012). The ACT approach encourages the client to respond to internal experiences (such as thoughts, images, feelings, and memories) as "events in the mind," rather than literal content, and helps the client develop a perspective of mindful acceptance toward them. This form of intervention can be particularly helpful when clients are struggling with internal events that are not amenable to control, or when persisting with efforts to control them leads to problems in everyday living. An aspect of the approach is to reduce the client's tendency to try to make literal sense of an experience when it is not useful; ACT helps the client notice when "making sense" of experiences functions as an unhelpful form of control that maintains difficulties. ACT facilitates a shift in emphasis for clients, from focusing on trying to control internal events to focusing more on behavior-change processes that can lead to positive outcomes.

ACT's treatment efficacy across a range of clinical disorders and problems is gaining empirical support (A-Tjak et al., 2015). Studies show that ACT performs better than either treatment as usual or active control interventions, and they indicate that ACT and established psychological treatments (usually CBT) achieve equivalent outcomes for several disorders. Division 12 of the American Psychological Association, Society of Clinical Psychology, states that there is "modest research support" for ACT as a psychological treatment for a number of mental health problems, including anxiety, depression, and psychosis (http://www.div12.org/psychological-treatments/treatments/acceptance-and-commitment-therapy-for-psychosis). Furthermore, studies suggest that ACT does appear to work through the processes suggested by the psychological flexibility model (Levin, Hildebrandt, Lillis, & Hayes, 2012).

The Psychological Flexibility Model

The six core theoretical processes of ACT are set out in the hexaflex model (figure 1), and they work together to increase *psychological flexibility*, defined as "the ability to contact the present moment more fully as a conscious human being, and to change or persist in behavior when doing so serves valued ends" (Hayes et al., 2006, p. 7). Although the six processes are represented as distinct in the model, they are highly interdependent, such that starting to use one process is likely to positively impact the others. More recently, these processes have been grouped into three sets of response style: open, aware, and active (Hayes, Villatte, Levin, & Hildebrandt, 2011; see table 1 for a summary of these processes).

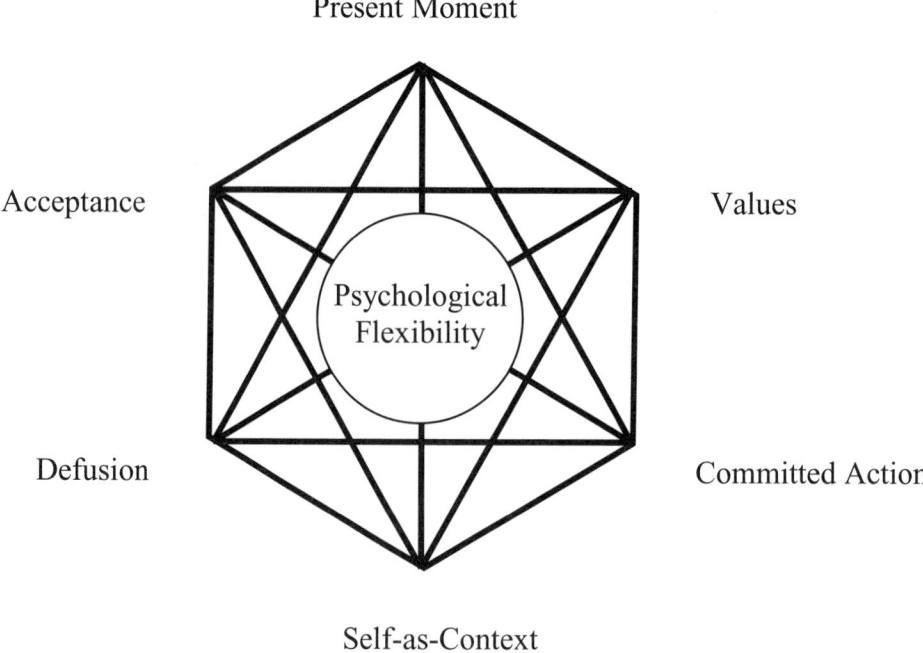

Figure 1. The ACT model of psychological flexibility, or hexaflex

Table 1. Central ACT processes

(adapted from Luoma, Hayes, & Walser, 2007)

Process	Definition
Open	
Acceptance	The active and aware embrace of psychological events (thoughts and emotions) without unnecessary attempts to change their frequency or form.
Defusion	The process of untangling from unhelpful thoughts and responding to mental experiences as experiences, rather than guides to action.
Aware	
Self-as-context	A continuous and secure "I" from which events are experienced, but that is also distinct from those events.
Present moment	Ongoing, nonjudgmental contact with internal (thoughts and emotions) and external events as they occur.
Active	
Values	Desired and chosen life directions.
Committed action	The process of linking specific actions to chosen values and building successively larger patterns of effective actions.

OPEN

The processes of acceptance and defusion work together to assist the broader skill of developing openness toward internal content (thoughts, emotions, memories). *Acceptance* is the process by which clients "embrace" their thoughts and feelings without trying to resist, avoid, or suppress them (experiential avoidance). This acceptance is not merely a passive process of tolerance or resignation but a full willingness to step toward and make space for psychological phenomena, including psychotic symptoms, without engaging in an unworkable struggle against them.

Alongside the process of acceptance, defusion further supports an open stance toward internal experience. Defusion exercises help clients "step back" from internal experiences, such as thoughts, memories, or appraisals of unusual experiences, and see them for what they are (experiences), rather than what they say they are (guides to action and choices), thereby reducing the literal rule-based responses to internal events that are unhelpful. From an ACT perspective, fusion increases the likelihood that an individual's behavioral repertoire will narrow in response to such experiences, thereby reducing opportunities for values-based actions. Defusion works to expand the repertoire by undermining one's entanglement with the thoughts and verbal rules that promote restriction or avoidance.

AWARE

Self-as-context refers to the sense of self (I, here, now), from which all internal experiences are observed and contained. An awareness of this particular perspective, cultivated through a mindful contact with the present moment, can loosen attachment to distressing thoughts, images, beliefs, or hallucinations that may arise. Mindfulness (present moment awareness) can help individuals learn to notice but not judge passing thoughts, feelings, or images in order to develop a more decentered stance toward internal experiences and to support engagement with core values.

ACTIVE

The heart of ACT work is assisting clients to become more engaged with and active in their lives in a chosen way. This happens through a process of identifying and constructing sets of values and then using them to inform the steps one takes toward meaningful goals and specific action plans. Goals are set in ways that increase the likelihood they will be met (for example, setting initially small, measurable tasks, which are increasingly built into larger patterns of committed action).

Mindfulness (Noticing) within ACT

It is worth including a little more detail on mindfulness and its use within ACT, given that the term is used in numerous contexts and, depending on personal experience and practice, is likely to mean different things to different readers. *Mindfulness* is generally described as "paying attention in a particular way: on purpose, in the present moment, and non-judgmentally" (Kabat-Zinn,

1994, pp. 3–4), wherein a person intentionally focuses attention on present-moment experiences in a nonjudgmental and accepting way, and also with compassion and curiosity toward these experiences (Kabat-Zinn, 2003). We can contrast this state of mind with engaging in cognitive processes such as rumination, worry, planning, and fantasizing, or behaving automatically without awareness—that is, being on autopilot (Baer, Smith, & Allen, 2004; K. W. Brown & Ryan, 2003).

Mindfulness has been a component of a number of cognitive behavioral therapy approaches, beginning with dialectical behavior therapy (DBT) for borderline personality disorder (Linehan, 1993). Mindfulness as practiced within mindfulness-based stress reduction (MBSR) was incorporated as a component of mindfulness-based cognitive therapy (MBCT) to help prevent further relapses in people with recurrent major depression (Segal, Williams, & Teasdale, 2002). One of the challenges to the practitioner's understanding of mindfulness is that, although we can learn how to use it as a technique, there are various definitions, including mindfulness as a psychological process, an outcome, or a collection of techniques (Hayes et al., 2012). Within MBCT, for example, the practice of mindfulness is seen as an alternative cognitive mode (Teasdale, 1999) that is incompatible with the kind of cognitive processing that increases risk for relapse in depression.

The rationale for mindfulness within ACT focuses on how it can promote flexible responding and taking action based upon chosen personal values. Mindfulness uses four processes from the psychological flexibility model: present-moment awareness, acceptance, defusion, and self-as-context (Fletcher & Hayes, 2005). This functional definition of mindfulness in ACT means that there is no linkage with particular mindfulness exercises or techniques, so any method that changes these processes is relevant (Hayes & Shenk, 2004).

ACT as a Recovery Therapy

ACT promotes recovery and social inclusion by shifting client focus from that of symptom control to connecting with personal values and participating in life as other people do and as the client may have in the past. The ACT approach maps nicely onto CHIME, the recovery processes mentioned earlier:

- **Connectedness:** The prosocial approach of ACT orients people to connect with others, to learn from their experiences, to understand their perspectives, and to develop compassion for oneself and others. It also helps us to appreciate that we can all step forward in our own journey of personal recovery and purpose.

- **Hope:** Maintaining hope is an active stance we can take on an ongoing basis. Also, while difficult thoughts and feelings may come and go, the hopeful actions that people take are tangible ways to make positive life changes.

- **Identity:** A positive identity can be reestablished by contacting with self-as-awareness and by noticing how our minds create stories about us. Instead of being entangled in the mind's judgments, we observe whether they are useful for our chosen life directions.

- **Meaning:** By finding meaning, we can dignify life's pain and suffering if they are part of the process of doing the things that are important to us. By acting on personal values, we can increase our contact with meaning.

- **Empowerment:** This involves self-management and taking responsibility for one's life. We help people to be "response-able": to act on their values, rather than their fear, through developing an open, compassionate stance toward their experiences and themselves, and by learning from experience.

The clear fit of ACT with recovery principles shows how contextual approaches can inform the way we offer help to people with serious mental illness. ACT assumes that people can develop psychological flexibility regardless of the presenting problem, including persisting psychotic symptoms.

Rationale for ACT for Psychosis (ACTp)

There are a number of reasons why an ACT approach can be useful for people experiencing and recovering from psychosis. Ultimately, improvements in functioning and quality of life result from changes in behavior rather than reductions in positive symptoms (Bach, 2004), and psychological flexibility can mediate these changes. In addition to increasing well-being, reducing avoidance, and enhancing values-based living, promoting psychological flexibility with ACT offers benefits for the particular problems and symptoms of psychosis. Some of the qualities (intrusive, uncontrollable, negative, frightening) of distressing voices and delusional beliefs increase the likelihood that people respond to them with suppression or avoidance (Morris, Garety, & Peters, 2014; Oliver, O'Connor, Jose, McLachlan, & Peters, 2012). Conversely, some psychotic experiences can be very engaging, in that they can be magical, interesting, and have high personal meaning, especially in the context of a life devoid of meaningful activity and social connection. As such, clients may engage with these experiences to escape a mundane life, although doing so has the potential for high personal cost in the long term. The qualities of positive psychotic symptoms and people's responses to them are discussed further below. In addition, people with psychosis can display particular reasoning biases that limit psychological flexibility, including a tendency to blame other people for negative events (Martin & Penn, 2002), a tendency to jump to conclusions on the basis of relatively little evidence (Dudley, Taylor, Wickham, & Hutton, 2015), and a poor ability to generate alternative explanations for experiences (Freeman et al., 2004).

RESPONDING TO VOICES

Auditory hallucinations tend to be compelling verbal experiences for people with psychosis, and they are often negative, personally salient, and highly distressing (Nayani & David, 1996). To try to cope, people who hear voices develop responses based on their beliefs about the voices and interpersonal beliefs about their social standing within relationships. People might resist or engage with voices, depending on whether they perceive the voices as malevolent or benevolent, respectively (Chadwick & Birchwood, 1995).

Resistance is an attempt to suppress or control voices, with the aim of eliminating or reducing them. Resistance to hostile voices can be divided into the fundamental *fight* (attempts to confront) or *flight* (attempts to escape or avoid) responses (P. Gilbert et al., 2001), coping methods that tend to be ineffective in the long run. Research has shown that fight strategies, such as shouting back at or arguing with voices, are associated with poorer emotion control (Farhall & Gehrke, 1997), and flight responses, such as trying to block out the voices, are associated with depression (Escher, Delespaul, Romme, Buiks, & van Os, 2003) and reduced self-esteem (Haddock, Slade, Bentall, Reid, & Faragher, 1998). Resistance strategies may also have the effect of maintaining voices and beliefs about their power and identity in the longer term (Morrison & Haddock, 1997). In terms of the fight response, actively hostile attitudes and behaviors toward voices can increase physiological arousal, which contributes to increased voice frequency (P. Gilbert et al., 2001; Romme & Escher, 1989). The flight response of engaging in safety-seeking behaviors, such as appeasing or complying with the commands of malevolent voices (done to prevent a feared outcome), prevents the disconfirmation of the person's fearful beliefs about the voices (Hacker, Birchwood, Tudway, Meaden, & Amphlett, 2008).

Engagement, on the other hand, is defined as "elective listening, willing compliance, and doing things to bring on the voices" (Chadwick & Birchwood,

1994, p. 192). It involves listening to some or all of the voices and directly accepting what they say (Farhall & Gehrke, 1997; Frederick & Cotanch, 1995). However, actively engaging with voices has the potential to become overly intimate and may have hidden costs in terms of flexibility, confidence, and engagement with other activities and relationships (Birchwood & Chadwick, 1997). Passive engagement may incorporate submissive responses to voices, such as complying with commands from benevolent voices (Braham, Trower, & Birchwood, 2004; Shawyer et al., 2008).

These forms of response—engagement and resistance—may inadvertently reinforce the experience of hearing voices and compound the client's distress and disability. Both forms of response perpetuate the relationship with voices by keeping clients involved with them, and this continued preoccupation can impede the pursuing of important life goals (for a more detailed discussion see Thomas, Morris, Shawyer, & Farhall, 2013).

DELUSIONAL THINKING

Experiences associated with delusional thinking, such as anxiety, shame, or humiliation, can directly lead people to avoid these experiences and triggering situations. This familiar form of experiential avoidance has been termed *passive* avoidance (García-Montes, Luciano Soriano, Hernández-López, & Zaldívar, 2004), whereby the person seeks to avoid private experiences and behaves in ways to reduce those experiences and the conditions that generate them. Some delusions, however, can be understood as *active* forms of experiential avoidance (García-Montes et al., 2004; García-Montes, Pérez-Álvarez, & Perona-Garcelán, 2013). With these, the experiential avoidance is more elaborate, and the delusional symptom itself becomes a means of avoiding some other matter (for example, low self-esteem, guilt, or depression). The "active" aspect of experiential avoidance overlaps with cognitive fusion, whereby the person verbally constructs an alternative reality or world, which they become fused with and immersed in via the processes of worry and rumination. Although, a person's delusions may not always start this way, these processes become maintaining factors. This overinvolvement with the content of delusions, while initially positively reinforcing, can have a negative impact on the person's valued life directions.

ACCEPTANCE APPROACHES

Given the negative impact that suppression and avoidance strategies have in the long term, acceptance is a potentially more adaptive response to psychotic experiences. Cohen and Berk (1985) identified acceptance as a "do nothing" coping response used by some patients with schizophrenia, suggesting they had learned to live with their symptoms. They distinguished this response from a less healthy "do nothing" strategy involving helplessness and giving up.

One way that therapists have attempted to promote acceptance in therapy has been to cultivate insight. This form of acceptance has been a part of some forms of cognitive behavioral therapy for psychosis (CBTp; Kingdon & Turkington, 1994). Interventions include nonconfrontational and personalized discussions of alternative models of experiences, including the evaluation of beliefs about the power and identity of voices or other perpetrators and, ultimately, the reattribution of unusual experiences to the self (Garety, Fowler, & Kuipers, 2000). By accepting symptoms as part of an illness rather than as coming from real people, therapists hope that people will be less fearful and will be able to disengage from the content of voices and beliefs (Chadwick & Birchwood, 1994; van der Gaag, 2006). However, such discussions within CBTp have the potential to be unhelpful if the therapist does not consider the function of the symptoms, particularly if they are forms of active avoidance as described above. It is also possible that, by excessively focusing on cognition and the search for meaning, and by communicating the need to "fix thinking" before effective action can be taken, some therapeutic efforts to modify thoughts may actually maintain or accentuate processes that impede recovery (Bach, 2004).

Romme and colleagues pioneered an important acceptance approach; they suggest that clients can learn to accept voices by exploring their personal meaning, acknowledging their positive aspects, and learning to incorporate them into life rather than attempting to eliminate them (Romme & Escher, 1989; Romme & Escher, 1993; Romme, Honig, Noorthoorn, & Escher, 1992). This work has been influential with groups for people who hear voices, such as Intervoice: The International Hearing Voices Network, and via self-help publications, peer-support groups, conferences, and online resources. More recently, this approach has been incorporated into a case-formulation intervention for voices, to help clients understand the meaning of voice content within the context of broader life experiences and interpersonal relationships (Longden, Corstens, Escher, & Romme, 2012), and to help them relate to voices in more accepting ways through voice dialogue (Corstens, Longden, & May, 2012).

Though quite different in approach, all these therapeutic forms of acceptance depend on the person "accepting" some particular explanation for psychotic experiences. Thus, interventions incorporating this approach rely on the person adhering to a verbally based narrative about the experience. It is assumed that these revised understandings will result in less distress and life disruption. While these client-formed explanations may inform the use of certain coping strategies, they do not specifically encompass skills to accept the presence of psychotic experiences as they occur. This is important, because the experiences of voices and other anomalous experiences in the moment often remain real and engulfing despite clients having the ability to reflect on them afterward. As a result, these alternative explanations and frameworks to promote acceptance may have limited effectiveness in those moments when clients need help the most.

An ACT Approach to Psychosis

ACT highlights a form of acceptance that fosters skills that people can apply as psychotic experiences occur. This mindful acceptance is neither a specific coping strategy nor a process of providing meaning, rather it's a particular style of relating to uncontrollable psychological events. It involves the skills of *nonjudgmental awareness*, deliberately observing mental events as they occur without judging them as good or bad and without reacting to them, and *disengagement* (detachment), detaching from the literal meaning of the content of voices and delusions—that is, distinguishing the actual experience (sounds and words) from what it represents (literal reality). (See the definition of "defusion" in table 1.)

The broader mindfulness and psychosis literature informs the mindful acceptance of psychotic experiences within ACT (Chadwick, Newman-Taylor, & Abba, 2005; Dannahy et al., 2011). For example, Chadwick's (2006) person-based cognitive therapy (PBCT) emphasizes the development of metacognitive awareness through mindfulness practice to reduce experiential avoidance and entanglement with psychotic experiences. Studies indicate that mindfulness-based interventions (MBIs) are acceptable and can be useful for people with distressing symptoms of psychosis (Chadwick et al., 2016; Khoury et al., 2013; Strauss, Thomas, & Hayward, 2015).

The therapeutic focus of ACT—changing the person's relationship with symptoms, rather than the symptoms themselves—can reduce the impact of the symptoms and help the person focus more on valued actions (Pérez-Álvarez, García-Montes, Perona-Garcelán, & Vallina-Fernández, 2008). ACT emphasizes the *workability* of the individual's behavior, with greater flexibility and more response options (Pankey & Hayes, 2003). For example, through acceptance work, a person who typically responds to hearing voices with social isolation and arguing with them may develop a broader range of behavioral responses to hearing voices. These might include activities, such as going out of the house, having a conversation with another person, deliberately noticing the acoustic properties of the voices, or engaging in a valued activity, as well as their usual responses to control the voices. The clinical focus of ACT is to add new positive functions and associations to the experience of hearing voices.

Evidence Base for ACTp

Five randomized controlled trials (RCTs) have evaluated the efficacy of ACT approaches for people with psychosis (Bach & Hayes, 2002; Gaudiano & Herbert, 2006; Shawyer et al., 2012; Shawyer et al., 2017; White et al., 2011), and there have been systematic reviews of these approaches for psychosis as well (Cramer, Lauche, Haller, Langhorst, & Dobos, 2016; Khoury et al., 2013; Ost, 2014). Although the trials had modest sample sizes, the findings were promising, indicating that such interventions may help reduce the impact of psychotic symptoms, particularly in terms of believability and emotional impact and disruption to functioning; they also had positive follow-up outcomes (Bach, Hayes, & Gallop, 2012). Importantly, all the studies showed that the interventions are feasible and acceptable with this group of people, and that it is possible for participants to respond in a psychologically flexible way to their unusual experiences. Clients do not get overwhelmed, provided that the mindfulness and other experiential exercises are adapted to take into account their difficulties.

The initial RCTs focused on rehospitalization rates. Bach and Hayes (2002) randomly allocated eighty inpatients with positive psychotic symptoms to treatment as usual (TAU) or to four individual sessions of ACT plus TAU. The ACT involved teaching patients to defuse from difficult thoughts, feelings, and psychotic experiences (just noticing them rather than treating them as true or false) and to identify and focus on actions directed toward valued goals. The ACT participants had lower rehospitalization rates than the TAU participants at the four-month follow-up, and this difference was maintained one-year postdischarge (Bach, Hayes, et al., 2012). There was an outcome difference worth noting; the intervention had little impact on the rehospitalization rate of participants with delusions but a large treatment effect for those experiencing auditory hallucinations.

In a smaller study comparing TAU and ACT plus TAU for psychotic inpatients, Gaudiano and Herbert (2006) found that, at discharge, patients in the ACT treatment arm showed greater improvements in mood, social impairment, and distress associated with hallucinations. Although the four-month rehospitalization rates were similar to those of the 2002 study, the group difference was not statistically significant.

RCTs involving outpatient psychosis samples have focused on either depression following psychosis or responses to ongoing positive symptoms. White and colleagues (2011) conducted an RCT of ACT for emotional dysfunction following psychosis, in which the participants were recovering from a recent episode of psychosis and experiencing depression or anxiety, or both. They compared a ten-session ACT intervention plus TAU (community psychiatric care) with TAU alone. Those receiving ACT showed a significant reduction in depression and negative symptoms, plus they had significantly fewer crisis contacts over the course of the study. White and colleagues recently completed the ADAPT study, a pilot RCT of ACT for depression after psychosis (ACTdp), comparing ACT plus standard care (SC) with SC alone, in order to inform a definitive, pragmatic multicenter trial of the effectiveness of ACTdp (Gumley et al., 2016).

The treatment of resistant command hallucinations (TORCH) trial compared befriending with fifteen sessions of an acceptance-enhanced CBT (A-CBT) intervention (Shawyer et al., 2012). There were no significant differences in the blind-rated outcome measures between the A-CBT and befriending groups (both interventions showed improvements), although the A-CBT participants reported subjectively greater improvement with command hallucinations. While the quality of the trial was high, it had difficulty recruiting the full number of participants with command hallucinations to have adequate power. The Lifengage trial (Thomas et al., 2014) compared eight sessions of ACT with befriending therapy for ninety-six outpatients with persisting and distressing psychotic symptoms. Participants in both therapy groups improved, and there was no group difference in overall mental state. However, participants in the ACT group were more satisfied with therapy and reported greater subjective benefit. They also showed greater improvement in positive symptoms at follow-up, consistent with the treatment focus in the study (Shawyer et al., 2017).

Mediation analyses within these treatment trials suggest that changing the targeted processes of psychological flexibility is what achieved the positive clinical effects of ACT for psychosis (ACTp). Changes in mindfulness mediated emotional adjustment to psychosis (White et al., 2011), and the reduced believability of hallucinations mediated the effect of ACT on hallucination-related distress (Gaudiano, Herbert, & Hayes, 2010). Using the combined data from the Bach and Hayes (2002) and Gaudiano and Herbert (2006) studies, Bach, Gaudiano, Hayes, and Herbert (2012) found that the decreased believability in the literal content of psychotic symptoms postintervention significantly mediated the effect of ACT on rehospitalization rates. Clinicians consider believability a proxy for cognitive defusion, and it has mediated ACT outcomes in other populations too (Zettle, Rains, & Hayes, 2011). In addition to mediation studies, qualitative data from client interviews have revealed similar themes with regard to the active therapeutic processes of ACTp: mindfulness, defusion, acceptance, and values work (Bacon, Farhall, & Fossey, 2014).

Adaptations to the Practice of ACT with People with Psychosis

In using ACT with people experiencing psychosis, it has been necessary to adapt interventions to suit the client group and service contexts. This section outlines some of these practical adaptations, drawn from our own experiences and those of others in the wider literature.

THERAPEUTIC RELATIONSHIP

The therapeutic relationship is a key part of any form of psychological intervention for psychosis. It has been highlighted as being central to cognitive behavioral therapy for psychosis (CBTp; for example, Johns, Jolley, Keen, & Peters, 2014), and research has found the therapeutic alliance to be causal in determining whether or not clients benefited from CBTp (Goldsmith, Lewis, Dunn, & Bentall, 2015). Within ACTp, the therapeutic relationship is validating, normalizing, and collaborative. It creates a context that teaches the limits of literal language for problem solving and encourages the experiential learning of different ways of relating to private experiences while expanding values-based behaviors.

The social context of the relationship involves *radical acceptance*, an appreciation of the whole person. In addition to the therapist accepting the client, radical acceptance includes clients accepting themselves, including unwanted experiences, and other people. The therapist views clients as complete human beings, not broken or different, for whom psychosis is one part. The therapist-client connection, with the common experience of being human, is nicely illustrated by the "two mountains" metaphor (Hayes, Strosahl, & Wilson, 1999), which therapists can share with clients when introducing ACT to them:

> It's like you're climbing your mountain over there and I am climbing my mountain over here. From where I am on my mountain I can see

things on your mountain that you can't see—I might be able to see an easier pathway, or that you're using your pickaxe incorrectly, or that there's an avalanche about to happen. But I wouldn't want you to think I'm sitting on the top of my mountain, no problems, no issues, just sitting back and enjoying life. I'm climbing my own mountain, over here. And we're all climbing our mountain till the day we die. But what we can learn to do is to climb more effectively, climb more efficiently, and learn how to enjoy the climbing. We can learn how to take a break and have a good rest and take in the view and appreciate how far we've come. We're both in the same boat, we're dealing with the human condition.

This metaphor highlights how we are in the same situation as those recovering from serious mental illness; we all face the challenge of living according to our values despite unwanted and entangling experiences. However, it is also important to acknowledge that people with psychosis often have a greater number of experiences (of greater intensity, too) to handle in their lives. We can end the metaphor with something like this: "I don't have to know anything about what it feels like to climb your mountain to see where you are about to step or to see what might be a better path for you to take." Facilitator self-disclosure—the ways they struggle and the between-session commitments they will undertake—is an important component of our ACTp groups. Not only does this modeling engage group participants, it encourages the sense of universality and perspective-taking described above.

OPEN PROCESSES

Acceptance and defusion work together to assist the broader skill of developing openness toward internal experiences. Clients are encouraged to embrace their thoughts and feelings without trying to resist, avoid, or suppress them. This form of acceptance is not a passive process of tolerance or resignation but a full willingness to have experiences (which can persist with psychosis despite treatment). The ACT emphasis on learning by addition (rather than replacement) is key for this client group, who often remain attached to coping strategies that are effective in modulating extremely distressing experiences in the short term. In the ACTp groups, it is useful to understand which strategies participants use in order to get things done in their lives, and to respectfully introduce the idea of willingness as an additional skill in the toolkit. Therapists encourage experiential learning, that clients "try willingness out" to see if the approach can result in more valued actions.

AWARE PROCESSES

When using mindfulness with people with psychosis, some adaptations are necessary to take into account experiences related to unpleasant voices, images, or paranoid thoughts (Chadwick et al., 2005). As in MBSR protocols, we start with breath and body awareness, using the breath as a central focal point. However, the breath focus is difficult for some clients with high anxiety or dissociative experiences, so it can be helpful to use the soles of the feet as the focal point, which helps to ground the person in the room. In our mindfulness practices, we invite participants to cultivate an ongoing awareness of psychotic experiences and the associated thoughts and feelings. The practices carefully limit states of deep concentration, which have been linked to the onset of auditory hallucinations (Chadwick, 2006), and we use briefer and more "talky" mindfulness exercises than those used in MBSR and MBCT. None of the mindfulness exercises is longer than ten minutes, so as not to be overwhelming to participants experiencing distressing symptoms. We give frequent instructions, with pauses of no longer than ten seconds in the initial exercises, in case participants find silence difficult and become lost in responses to psychotic experiences. Pauses are extended slightly during exercises in the latter sessions. The mindfulness exercises are termed "noticing" exercises and include a range of practices, including mindful eating, stretching, and walking. We encourage home practice, supported by audio recordings of the exercises used in the workshops, but take an accepting stance to noncompletion.

As with any mindfulness exercise, the debrief inquiry about what participants notice is often the most challenging stage. This is particularly the case with this group of clients, who are very focused on developing methods to further control their experiences and can be quick to notice the immediate benefits of the exercises, such as relaxation. We aim to balance the need to reinforce the range of experiences that participants notice, both positive and negative, with any response that highlights ACT-consistent processes. We gently emphasize these processes to the rest of the group and also model them in our feedback.

ACTIVE PROCESSES

Identifying and clarifying values in this client group, particularly for those individuals with established psychosis, can bring up themes of loss and missed opportunities. Some participants might be unclear of what they value, especially if they have personal histories of invalidation or trauma, or participants may have lost touch with their values through channeling their efforts to manage the psychosis. Although people's experiences of the past impact the group work, as well as the ways people can act more effectively in the present, ACTp focuses less on the past and more on the idea of constructing a meaningful life, starting from today. Connecting with values is seen as a work in progress and as a voyage of discovery, a trying out of new things. We sometimes describe it like fashion and trying on new clothes—unfamiliar and uncomfortable to begin with but getting more comfortable with time. In line with other authors, we also highlight compassion to self and others as a valued life direction (White, 2015).

Committed action is an integral part of the therapy. In ACTp workshops, we encourage clients to set values-based goals by identifying a small action in line with their values that they can complete between sessions. We emphasize that completion is not the only aim of the committed action; the ability to notice thoughts, emotions, and sensations that may show up along the way and, crucially, automatic and unhelpful responses to these, are also important processes. The process of "setting" homework was influenced by previous research on engaging people in behavioral activation: dividing into smaller groups, providing plenty of reinforcement for small steps, and understanding the balance between control and willingness that is needed to manage having intense experiences.

THERAPEUTIC STYLE

As with CBTp, ACTp is matched to the client's pace, and it has a gentle, conversational style. The use of scaffolding is important in our workshops; facilitators model and use examples, thus enabling clients to build up to applying the exercises themselves. Showing videos and case vignettes can also make it easier for participants to share their experiences, ways of coping, and values. Experiential and physicalizing exercises are used as much as possible to bring the therapy alive and to make the learning points more memorable. We act out our central metaphor, the "passengers on the bus," so that participants can experiment in session with how to relate differently to distressing thought content.

ACT Groups for People with Psychosis (G-ACTp)

There are a number of motives for developing ACT as a group-based intervention for people who experience psychosis (G-ACTp; for further discussion, see McArthur, Mitchell, & Johns, 2013). The explicit sharing of common human experience and the underlying transdiagnostic model of ACT both suit group delivery (Hayes et al., 2011; Walser & Pistorello, 2004). In addition, particular aspects of the intervention lend themselves to a group format: many ACT metaphors are interactive and benefit from more people, observing others being present and willing can promote these processes in oneself, and making commitments in a social context is likely to strengthen action. For people with psychosis, group interventions can be particularly valuable, affording opportunities for normalizing psychotic experiences, gaining peer support, and facilitating perspective-taking skills, all of which augment specific therapeutic strategies (Abba, Chadwick, & Stevenson, 2008; Dannahy et al., 2011; Jacobsen, Morris, Johns, & Hodkinson, 2011; Ruddle, Mason, & Wykes, 2011). Our workshops aim to connect participants and facilitators around our shared humanity, help reduce stigma, and increase self-compassion. We also validate the courage participants show in expanding their lives despite the difficulties associated with psychosis, including fearing recurrence, wanting to appease voices, being concerned about the motives of other people, and coping with social stressors.

In terms of the therapist-client ratio and/or number of group sessions offered, group interventions can be a more efficient use of therapist time than individual work. Mental health staff from different professional groups can be trained via workshops to facilitate group-based interventions (Oliver, Venter, & Lloyd, 2014; Wykes et al., 2005). In addition, groups offer staff excellent opportunities for development through cofacilitation. Hence, brief group ACT (G-ACT) formats, which can be readily disseminated through staff training, offer the potential for cost-effective, wide-scale delivery.

Development of the ACT for Recovery Group Intervention and Manual

Our G-ACTp intervention evolved from efforts to develop therapeutic groups that would engage clients with psychosis living in inner-city boroughs of South London. Considering the difficulties in accessing individual CBTp and the benefits of group approaches, G-ACTp offered promise by expanding the choice and availability of psychological therapies. The intervention seemed applicable and helpful for a diverse set of mental health service users from different cultural and socioeconomic backgrounds.

We developed our treatment manual for community and inpatient settings over several years, drawing on brief ACT interventions to reduce psychotic relapse and on mindfulness groups for people with psychosis. We piloted it in early intervention and community psychosis teams and further adapted it for inpatient wards (described in chapter 3). Influenced by our local context, it seemed important to make the groups welcoming, fun, and lighthearted. However, there were many heartfelt moments when group members shared their courage in committing to values-based actions or connected with how challenging it can be to experience and recover from psychosis.

ACT FOR LIFE STUDY

We formally evaluated our G-ACTp intervention in the ACT for Life study (reported by Johns et al., 2015). The first aim of this study was to determine the feasibility and acceptability of delivering the intervention, according to a standardized, manualized protocol, in routine community psychosis services in the United Kingdom. The second aim was to conduct a preliminary evaluation of clinical outcomes that could inform the future development of the intervention and randomized controlled evaluation. The ACT for Life study found that our four-week G-ACTp intervention was feasible for and acceptable to people with psychosis. Uncontrolled pre- and postassessments suggested that participants experienced small improvements in mood and functioning, as well as changes in their psychological flexibility processes consistent with the ACT model.

We were successful in our manualization of the intervention, and it was possible to deliver G-ACTp using a standardized protocol in a routine service setting. (You can download the *ACT for Life* manual at http://drericmorris.com/wp-content/uploads/2014/10/ACT-for-Life-Groups-Manual-2012.pdf, and further details of the study and the ACT for recovery group protocol are also described by Butler and colleagues, 2016.) We chose a brief group format (four two-hour sessions, held weekly), partly based on the research literature but also on our experience; we understood the challenges of running longer therapy groups and maintaining consistent attendance over a number of weeks. The group was closed, comprising four to eight participants, and facilitated by a lead therapist competent in ACT who was accompanied by one or two cofacilitators, mental health practitioners with experience working with people with psychosis. They had also attended a two-day ACT training designed for the study. The two-hour workshop sessions were structured to make the experience predictable each week, and every session had a similar format: a warm-up exercise, two noticing (mindfulness) exercises, a review of the committed action, a group discussion and activity (including role-playing and experiential exercises), time to plan a committed action for the coming week, and feedback.

We used experiential exercises as much as possible to highlight the processes by which participants can become caught up in struggling with their symptoms and adopt ineffective ways of coping. Exercises were brief and learning points were carefully paced and structured to accommodate any cognitive difficulties. Drawing on participant feedback from our previous pilot work, we chose the "passengers on the bus" metaphor (Hayes et al., 1999) as the central, overarching theme for the workshop sessions. The sessions were all supplemented by PowerPoint slides, worksheets, audio recordings of the mindfulness exercises, and handouts summarizing group content. We paid particular attention to supporting practice between sessions. At the close of each session, participants described the committed actions they were going to undertake during the week, which we reviewed in the following session. We offered an optional midweek telephone reminder for this action. This "check in" phone call reinforced any noticing of internal experiences participants had while they tried to engage in committed actions, and it also served as a reminder of the psychological flexibility skills covered in session. Participants also received a follow-up phone call two weeks after the final session. To further generalize the use of the skills in daily life, we encouraged participants to link up with their clinical team for continued support, and we gave them information about local activities and organizations.

The decision to use the passengers on the bus as the central metaphor proved to be successful. This metaphor describes driving your "bus of life," in which you, the bus driver, make choices about the direction your bus travels, moving toward or away from chosen values. On the bus are various passengers you have picked up on your journey of life, and they represent internal experiences (thoughts, feelings, memories, and sensations). The metaphor highlights the ways you interact with your passengers (for example, trying to get rid of them, agreeing with them, appeasing them, just noticing them) and how these interactions can limit or increase your movement in valued directions. All six ACT processes are represented within the metaphor, making it particularly beneficial, and it is applicable to all group members and facilitators.

In our G-ACTp protocol, we revisited the metaphor during each session and used it as a memory aid, which was helpful for participants who might otherwise struggle to recall the key elements. Initially we presented it as a story, and facilitators and participants later acted it out. We used a scripted video of a character describing challenges in his life, played by an actor, to illustrate the relevance and applicability of the metaphor. For participants experiencing auditory hallucinations, a potential issue that can arise is whether the hallucinated voice should act as a passenger. Given that most participants identified the voice as an external experience coming from an outside source, over which they had little control, we tended to encourage participants to label their thoughts and beliefs about the voice as the passengers. However, for clients who understand that their voices are self-generated, it is also possible to label the voice-hearing experience as a passenger.

ACT FOR RECOVERY STUDY

Based on the observations and outcomes of the ACT for Life study, the ACT for Recovery study developed the G-ACTp intervention further. For the evaluation study, we recruited clients with established psychosis, mainly due to service-development priorities and our clinical commitments. We also added G-ACT for caregivers as part of the intervention, which the generic exercise-based nature of our protocol allows us to do. We ran separate workshops for caregivers based on the same protocol (see chapter 2 for details). We feel it is important to consider the needs of caregivers, given that many service users maintain close contact with informal caregivers, and the caregiving role can have a negative and long-term impact on the mental and physical well-being of caregivers (Onwumere et al., 2015; Poon, Harvey, Mackinnon, & Joubert, 2016). It is well recognized that caring relationships are important for client recovery, and this fact has informed treatment recommendations for supporting caregivers themselves (for example, National Institute for Health and Care Excellence, 2014).

In ACT for recovery, we label the group sessions as "workshops" in the manual, both to emphasize the recovery-focus and skills-building aspects and to make the sessions relevant for caregivers, many of whom do not need to attend "therapy" groups. We also added an introductory "taster" session in which we introduce ACT principles and exercises; this allows people to opt in to the four-week course. This session helps reduce the chances of drop out after the first workshop session, which we observed in the ACT for Life study. Additionally, we run two weekly "booster" sessions, held eight weeks after the workshop program ends. These sessions do not introduce any new material; rather their aim is to provide a refresher of skills practiced in the sessions, and the opportunity for participants to reflect on any progress or difficulties encountered after the workshops have ended.

The sessions themselves retain the same structure and content, with minor adaptations to some of the exercises to improve participant understanding of the principles. We recorded videos specific for the workshops, one of an actor role-playing a client with psychosis (Paul), and one of an actor role-playing the client's caregiver (his father, George). We created an animation of the "passengers on the bus" metaphor, which provides a visual representation. As before, the workshops are facilitated by a lead therapist competent in ACT, accompanied by one or two cofacilitators who are either mental health practitioners or, novel to this intervention, service-user peer supporters. In updating the protocol, we thought that having experts by experience, those who have experienced mental health difficulties firsthand, would help to engage participants and add a dimension of validity in our efforts to link ACT processes to the journey of personal recovery within and beyond mental health services. In chapter 4 we describe this involvement of workshop cofacilitators with lived experience of mental health problems.

A pilot study, in which service users and caregivers either received G-ACTp immediately or after a twelve-week waiting period, evaluated the effectiveness of this intervention in improving well-being (Jolley et al., in press). Preliminary findings suggest that G-ACTp improves self-reported overall well-being, with no difference in outcomes immediately after the intervention, at twelve weeks, or between service users and caregivers.

Summary

Psychosis is a severe mental illness associated with reduced quality of life for both sufferers and family members. Cognitive behavioral therapy is recommended for people with psychosis, but access remains limited in front-line services. Group-based cognitive behavioral interventions, including ACT, have the potential to improve both the access and dissemination of therapy. ACT is a contextual cognitive behavioral intervention that lends itself to brief group therapy and to the diverse presentations of psychosis. This therapeutic approach emphasizes clients' relationship with their symptoms, helping them develop a perspective of mindful acceptance toward them, and encourages values-based living. The evidence base for ACT is growing across a range of physical and mental health problems, including psychosis. The key ACT processes work together to improve a person's psychological flexibility, and this approach can be particularly useful for people experiencing psychosis due to the qualities of psychotic symptoms and associated cognitive biases. ACT fosters mindful acceptance skills that can be applied as the psychotic experiences occur, and it helps the client focus less on symptoms and more on engaging in valued actions.

Our team has developed and adapted our approach to G-ACTp to suit the client group, and we have evaluated the groups in a range of community and inpatient settings. We wish to share our experience and learning in this area, so that you can run engaging and effective groups in your service context.

CHAPTER 2

Adapting ACT Workshops for Caregivers of People with Psychosis

Written with Suzanne Jolley

This chapter outlines our experiences offering ACT for recovery workshops for those who care for people with psychosis. We highlight the benefits of supporting these caregivers in psychosis settings and introduce the reservoir metaphor that we use in caregiver workshops. We then describe the adaptations we've made for the caregiver workshops and discuss helpful observations and suggestions gained from our experience facilitating them. And finally, we summarize qualitative and quantitative results from the caregiver workshops of the ACT for Recovery study.

"It Hurts to Care"—Caring for People with Serious Mental Illness

As outlined in chapter 1, the impact of psychosis can be both far-reaching and enduring, affecting not only individuals suffering from psychosis but also their loved ones and support systems. People experiencing psychosis often rely significantly on the unpaid contribution of family members, friends, and relatives, who help them meet their health and social care needs. These informal caregivers play an integral role in the recovery process of clients with psychosis (Lester et al., 2011; Pharoah, Mari, Rathbone, & Wong, 2010).

An informal caregiver is "someone who without payment provides help or support to a partner, child, relative, friend or neighbor who could not manage without their help" (Carers Trust, 2015), or, alternatively, an unpaid person who helps an individual cope with an illness or health condition (Hileman, Lackey, & Hassanein, 1992).

Many individuals with psychosis live with or remain in close contact with informal caregivers, often family members, and most commonly parents or partners (Lauber, Eichenberger, Luginbühl, Keller, & Rössler, 2003). Caregivers tend to be the main source of social contact for people with psychosis (Albert, Becker, McCrone, & Thornicroft, 1998). They often take an active role supporting their loved ones' psychosis recovery by identifying early signs of relapse, by encouraging them to take medication, and by making links with and helping them to access clinical services (Onwumere, Shiers, & Chew-Graham, 2016).

The Importance of Caring Relationships

Having caregiver support is helpful for people with psychosis, with research suggesting that clients who have access to a caring support system experience better outcomes, including fewer hospital admissions, shorter inpatient stays, and improved quality of life (Norman et al., 2005; Schofield, Quinn, Haddock, & Barrowclough, 2001), and they can derive greater gains from psychological therapies (Garety et al., 2008). Many caregivers describe their caring roles as satisfying and rewarding (Hsiao & Tsai, 2014; Lavis, 2015), and, importantly, clients themselves often express a desire for their caregivers to be involved in their care (Askey, Holmshaw, Gamble, & Gray, 2009; Walsh & Boyle, 2009). Caregivers are not only beneficial for client outcomes, but also cost effective. In the United Kingdom alone, it is estimated that the unpaid care of informal caregivers saves the public purse approximately £1.25 billion per year ($1.6 billion; Schizophrenia Commission, 2012).

The Challenges of Caregiving

Although caregiving can be rewarding for some, there is evidence that the role can have detrimental effects on the mental well-being and physical health of caregivers (Kuipers, Onwumere, & Bebbington, 2010). For example, many who care for people with psychosis experience clinical levels of depression, anxiety, trauma, stress, and physical ill-health (Barton & Jackson, 2008; S. Brown & Birtwistle, 1998; Kuipers et al., 2010; Laidlaw, Coverdale, Falloon, & Kydd, 2002). Such challenges can impact their abilities to cope with the demands placed upon them, particularly during times of mental health crisis (Lauber et al., 2003). Furthermore, caregivers often express feelings of shame, guilt, anger, and loss about the people they care for and about their own changing roles (Patterson, Birchwood, & Cochrane, 2005; Schene, van Wijngaarden, & Koeter, 1998).

Mental Health Services Find It Challenging to Support Caregivers

Much of the research literature on caring relationships in psychosis has focused on the construct of expressed emotion, which is considered an important measure of the caring environment. Expressed emotion is rated as high or low. Higher expressed emotion, characterized by emotional overinvolvement, hostility, and criticism on the part of a caregiver and/or family member, predicts more client relapses and hospital admissions for individuals with psychosis (Bebbington & Kuipers, 1994; Cechnicki, Bielańska, Hanuszkiewicz, & Daren, 2013). Conversely, low expressed emotion, characterized by positive family interactions, such as expressing warmth, can reduce the risk of relapse (Bebbington & Kuipers, 1994; Lee, Barrowclough, & Lobban, 2014).

Recent government policies have started to address the importance of responding to the needs of caregivers. For example, the UK National Institute for Health and Care Excellence (2014) and Royal Australian and New Zealand College of Psychiatrists (Galletly et al., 2016) suggest that caregiver-focused interventions, such as family interventions and educational and support programs, be offered to caregivers as early as possible.

Such recommendations are supported by research findings, which identify psychoeducation interventions as being consistently effective in improving the knowledge of caregivers, as well as their ability to cope with the demands of their roles (Sin & Norman, 2013). Family interventions have been shown to improve client outcomes by reducing expressed emotion and client relapse rates (Butzlaff & Hooley, 1998). In addition, family interventions have had positive effects on caregiver outcomes across Europe, Asia, and Australia, including reduced burden, improved distress levels (Giron et al., 2010), and greater satisfaction with services, as well as client outcomes, such as their perception of having support from caregivers (Kulhara, Chakrabarti, Avasthi, Sharma, & Sharma, 2009).

Despite the recommendations and recognized evidence base for family and caregiver interventions, structured treatments are not widely available or routinely offered in the United Kingdom (Berry & Haddock, 2008; Prytys, Garety, Jolley, Onwumere, & Craig, 2011) or the United States (Glynn, 2012). Often there are barriers that prevent mental health services from offering more support to caregivers, including organizational issues, lack of specialist training, and lack of supervision access (Onwumere, Grice, & Kuipers, 2016).

The Evidence Base of ACT for Caregivers

Several trials of ACT interventions have shown promising results for a range of formal and informal caregivers in different clinical populations. For example, ACT interventions have been offered to caregivers who face the stress and burden of caring for people with complex and enduring difficulties, including dementia (Losada et al., 2015), children with autism (Blackledge & Hayes, 2006), adolescents with anorexia nervosa (Merwin, Zucker, & Timko, 2013), individuals with acquired brain injuries (J. Williams, Vaughan, Huws, & Hastings, 2014), and people with intellectual disabilities and challenging behavior (Ingham, Riley, Nevin, Evans, & Gair, 2013; Noone & Hastings, 2010). All these studies identified significant improvements in caregiver well-being and level of burden following ACT interventions, and they highlight that ACT approaches are feasible for and acceptable to caregiver groups.

In their study assessing an eight-session ACT intervention aimed at reducing depression and anxiety symptoms in people caring for dementia sufferers, Losada and colleagues (2015) found that their intervention helped caregivers accept distressing internal events related to caregiving and to commit to and take action toward their values. They also noted that, by using acceptance coping strategies, caregivers decreased their levels of experiential avoidance in response to anxiety symptoms. Similarly, Blackledge and Hayes (2006) found that a two-day (fourteen-hour) workshop for parents of children recently diagnosed with autism showed promise in helping parents adjust to the difficulties of raising a child with autism. The authors suggested the ACT intervention reduced levels of experiential avoidance and cognitive fusion, which, they argued, played a role in reducing levels of general distress and depression in the parents.

Research has also explored the role of psychological flexibility in parents who are caregivers (Brassell et al., 2016; K. E. Williams, Ciarrochi, & Heaven, 2012). Greater psychological flexibility in parents is related to better outcomes, such as lower psychological distress (for example, distressing thoughts and feelings) and lower externalizing behaviors (for example, behavioral difficulties) in children and adolescents.

The Role of Psychological Flexibility in Caring

By describing psychologically inflexible responses, the opposite of flexible responses, we can use the psychological flexibility model (described in chapter 1) to understand how caring for a person with psychosis can be distressing and can affect the caregiver's quality of life.

Experiential avoidance (rather than acceptance or contact with the present moment): This can occur when caregivers are unwilling to be in contact with feelings, thoughts, and urges that arise from naturally challenging moments involved with caring. These psychologically inflexible responses could involve concern, frustration, conflicted ideas over what may be best to do, or anxiety about choices to increase the independence of the person they care for. Research has found that experientially avoidant coping strategies predict greater burnout and work-related stress in staff members who care for people with intellectual disabilities (Noone & Hastings, 2010).

In our ACT for recovery workshops, caregivers describe several examples of experiential avoidance, including withdrawing from a loved one in order to avoid uncomfortable thoughts or feelings about the person's situations or symptoms. They also describe actively avoiding addressing issues or potential confrontations with the people they care for by giving in to certain demands, such as providing money or overcompensating for loved ones by completing tasks of daily living that they know the people can complete themselves.

Cognitive fusion (rather than defusion or self-as-context): This can occur when the caregiver "buys in" to thoughts about the caring role in ways that lead to inflexibility and struggle. Cognitive fusion can occur when the caregiver feels shame, guilt, self-blame, or worry to such an extent that they feel increased distress, avoid rewarding moments, or have difficulty adapting to changes the person with psychosis displays. Cognitive fusion can also manifest when the caregiver feels engulfed or trapped by the caring role. We often witness caregivers expressing extreme guilt and self-blame regarding their loved one's difficulties. This has been particularly noticeable with parents.

Disconnection from values (rather than commitment to values): Caregivers sometimes sacrifice their connection with valued directions. We have witnessed caregivers experience great conflict regarding their values of caring versus maintaining their own well-being. Caregivers commonly describe reducing their social contacts, stopping hobbies and exercise, and, in extreme cases, giving up work in order to dedicate more time to caring for a loved one. When we encourage committed actions within workshops, caregivers sometimes express concern and feelings of guilt for spending time on themselves and not a loved one.

We feel that a brief intervention that focuses on strengthening caregivers' motivation to activate themselves based on personal values, and to step back from unwanted feelings and thoughts, allows them to be more in the moment in daily life and increases caregiver well-being.

Caregivers ACT for Recovery Workshops

We developed ACT for recovery workshops to address the psychological needs of people caring for individuals with psychosis. We were influenced by the promising results of ACT interventions for caregivers in various health settings, and our research study aimed to investigate how effectively brief ACT workshops could improve caregiver well-being in community psychosis settings.

As discussed in chapter 1, we describe the group sessions as "workshops" to emphasize the recovery focus and skills-building aspect of the intervention. The term also implies that caregivers do not have to consider themselves in need of psychological support in order to engage in the intervention. Due to the transdiagnostic nature of ACT, we offer the same protocol in workshops for both clients and caregivers, except for a few minor adjustments, discussed below. However, although the content of the group protocol remains similar, the ways in which participants and facilitators process and discuss the material tends to vary according to the different issues caregivers bring to the workshops.

Adapting ACT for Recovery Workshops for Caregivers

Below we discuss specific adaptations and suggestions that we feel may be pertinent to running ACT for recovery workshops with people who care for individuals with psychosis.

Recruitment

We have found that, at times, recruiting caregivers for workshops can be challenging. For example, many caregivers decline to attend when they find out that the workshops aren't about teaching them how to be "better caregivers" or offering them skills they can use to better support their loved ones experiencing psychosis. Feedback routinely indicates that caregivers do not feel they require or deserve psychological support, and many feel indulgent and guilty for participating in an intervention focused on their own well-being, as opposed to one that focuses on their loved one. We overcome such issues by discussing the reservoir metaphor (see below), which we use as a rationale to help caregivers understand that addressing their own needs and well-being is an important part of their caring roles.

In order to advertise caregiver workshops, we have developed posters and leaflets that acknowledge the vital role caregivers play in caring for people with psychosis. These materials highlight that we want to ensure that they are supported in their roles. The leaflets and posters also describe ACT, highlighting that the aim of the workshops is to encourage people to pursue what really matters to them while responding to difficult thoughts and feelings that might get in the way of what's important.

It is helpful if facilitators initially discuss with potential participants the content of the workshops, answering any queries they may have. Speaking directly to caregivers by phone or face-to-face can assist with engagement, especially if caregivers are nervous about attending a group focused on their own well-being. As with the client workshops, we believe it is necessary to invite potential caregiver participants to an introductory, or taster, session (see chapter 1 and part 2).

We have recruited participants from the clinical services where the research study was based, the South London and Maudsley NHS Foundation Trust. We offer the workshops to any caregivers of clients within the area's psychosis services, and we do not feel it necessary that their loved one also attends the client ACT for recovery workshops.

Caregiver-Only Workshops

We offer separate client and caregiver workshops. Despite the ACT approach being transdiagnostic, with the goal of improving well-being of both clients with psychosis and their caregivers, we believe that caregivers benefit from discussing their challenges of caring alongside people in similar positions, and we want them to feel that they are able to express themselves in a safe, open environment. For similar reasons, in cases where there are two identified caregivers from the same family, such as parents, we make the decision to invite them to separate caregiver workshops. We believe that if a couple were present in a workshop it might change the dynamic for other workshop participants. However, this may not be an issue in other settings.

Introducing the Reservoir Metaphor

During the taster and first sessions we introduce the reservoir metaphor (Kroeker, 2009) as a way of highlighting the important but often draining role of being a caregiver for someone experiencing psychosis:

We all have emotional reservoirs of different types. Some supply energy, others supply calmness, happiness, or well-being. When the reservoirs are full, we can maintain our energy, calmness, happiness, or well-being, even in times of stress, and we can carry on doing what's important in our lives. If there is a drought (such as a bad day or week, or other forms of stress), we maintain a healthy state because there is a supply in our reservoir.

We know that sometimes being a caregiver can be difficult and challenging, and this can drain one's reservoirs. If the reservoirs are dry, we are vulnerable to stresses: there may be some energy or happiness, but only if daily events are going well. The combination of dry reservoirs and a bad day can be problematic, and it may lead to difficulties, such as an emotional crash, lost temper, frustration, and so on.

The metaphor highlights the need to *replenish* one's reservoirs in order to continue serving in a caring role. We find that this metaphor often helps caregivers justify their workshop attendance and emphasizes the importance of their very challenging caring roles. Introducing the metaphor early in the workshops allows facilitators to reference it when caregivers bring up themes of guilt or self-indulgence about attending to their own values. These themes often arise during committed action exercises; rather than focusing on their own well-being, many caregivers report difficulty identifying a committed action that is not directly related to providing care for their loved one.

Here's an example of a time when we reiterated the reservoir metaphor in a workshop. A parent had identified the value of maintaining her physical health following a period of health complications. She identified goals relating to physical exercise, such as going for a walk or a bike ride. She reported that the client she cared for (her son) was unhappy about her spending time away, and that he felt her continued ill-health was good because it meant she had to stay at home with him rather than go to work. The caregiver felt guilty for wanting to improve her physical health and for spending time away from her son. By referring to the reservoir metaphor we highlighted that, by spending a specific amount of time on exercise, she was maintaining her physical health (thus, replenishing her reservoir), which would ensure that she could fulfill her demanding caring role.

The reservoir metaphor can help you suggest to caregivers that the aim of the workshops is to teach them different ways to maintain, or replenish, their reservoirs, which promotes well-being and helps them be capable of doing more of what's important in life.

Summarizing the Results from the ACT for Recovery Study

Below we briefly summarize the results of the ACT for Recovery study in relation to the caregiver participants.

Brief ACT Workshops Can Improve the Well-Being of Caregivers

Our ACT for Recovery study involved fifty-two caregivers of people with psychosis. They either received ACT for recovery group sessions immediately or after a twelve-week waiting period. The main outcome measure was self-reported well-being, rated at the start of the workshops (baseline, or zero weeks), posttreatment (at four weeks), and after two booster sessions (follow-up at twelve weeks). Caregivers who attended the workshops immediately reported improved overall well-being compared to the wait-list participants. These well-being improvements were maintained three months later. Both psychological flexibility and mindfulness improved over the course of the workshops for those who attended immediately. In looking at the outcomes of our workshops, we think that brief ACT interventions are beneficial in improving well-being for caregivers of people with psychosis.

Feedback from Caregivers

Besides assessing for well-being, psychological flexibility, and mindfulness, we also conducted interviews to gather specific feedback from several caregivers after they completed the workshops. They identified several positive experiences from the workshops.

OVERALL FEEDBACK ABOUT THE WORKSHOPS

Many caregivers said that attending the workshops improved their mood and psychological well-being. One stated, "My well-being is definitely improved. I'm less worried and anxious about what I'm doing."

Two participants reported that the workshops had additional benefits for their physical health. One said, "I've been quite physically unwell recently, but I'm managing it better now with the skills I learnt in the workshops." This improvement may be related to the fact that such caregivers started to attend to their own needs more, which may be linked to a reduction in distress and subsequent improvement in physical health. (However, this is just a hypothesis, as we did not directly test physical health in the study.)

REFLECTIONS ON MINDFULNESS (NOTICING) EXERCISES

Caregiver participants talked about increased self-awareness and ability to be more reflective, particularly as a result of the noticing exercises. For example, they reported that the noticing exercises allowed them to view things differently, to relax, and to respond differently to difficult internal experiences:

I'm trying to bring mindfulness into my routine, and I feel this has really helped with noticing how I feel.

The noticing exercises induced a sense of calm reflection.

Awareness helped me focus and think of the things that I want to achieve in my life.

Having never practiced noticing exercises before, many caregivers appeared somewhat nervous when we introduced the initial noticing exercise. We found it helpful to provide a justification for why we used noticing exercises, explaining the concept of automatic pilot and how noticing can be a way to direct one's attention to the present moment. We explained that we would guide them through the noticing exercise, which would last approximately five to ten minutes. We asked them to close their eyes, unless they preferred not to; if so, we asked them to focus on a spot in front of them. We then highlighted how natural it is for one's attention to wander, that it might happen repeatedly, and that we were interested in what they noticed. After the exercise, we discussed what they noticed, and facilitators modeled ACT-consistent responses (see chapter 5 for more discussion) for what the participants noticed during the exercise.

CONNECTING WITH VALUES

Alongside the benefits of the noticing exercises that caregivers identified, several participants expressed how the workshops helped them connect with their values and instilled in them the motivation to move toward their goals. Here are reflections from two participants:

The workshops gave me the platform to think and reflect on what is important in my life.

They've helped me set long-term goals…helped me find my purpose in life again.

Caregivers also reflected that initially they had difficulty identifying what was important and understanding the concept of values in their feedback. Many participants reported that setting values-related committed actions at the end of each session was a particularly important exercise. However, several identified a conflict between the caregiving role and pursuing their own valued goals, as noted by one participant:

If I follow my goals, I won't be able to be there for my daughter, which is my central dilemma…the trade-off between being available and pursuing my own career goals.

We will discuss how we addressed such conflicts later in the chapter.

PASSENGERS ON THE BUS METAPHOR

The "passengers on the bus" is the central metaphor we used in both the caregiver and client ACT for recovery workshops. Most caregiver participants found the metaphor useful. They particularly liked the "acting out the passengers on the bus" exercise (see part 2 for how to do this exercise), as it highlighted the different ways that people tend to respond to their passengers (for example, fight and struggle, give in, or respond with willingness) and the benefits and consequences of particular responses. Some caregivers said that the metaphor provided them greater awareness of their own passengers, and the process of externalizing and naming difficult internal experiences as "passengers" was helpful. Many also stated that the exercise provided a different way to respond to difficult passengers and allowed them more control over their lives. Here's what one participant said:

It's not a bad thing having passengers. I just need to accept them. Accept that I am a worrier, without letting it stop me. Don't feel guilty anymore. Make peace with myself. Accept passengers and allow them back on the bus. I can only be who I am. Accept myself and the good things I've done in life.

GROUP PROCESSES

One particularly noteworthy theme that emerged from the caregiver workshops relates to group processes in general. All interviewed caregivers reported benefits from merely being given the opportunity, time, and space to reflect with other people in the same caregiving position. Some stated that hearing from other caregivers who had experienced similar challenges and overcome difficulties that can occur in the caring role was validating and reassuring. Others reported that the workshops provided a supportive outlet for them to off-load their feelings.

Considerations for Engaging Caregivers in ACT Workshops

While facilitating ACT for recovery workshops for caregivers, we identified several issues that may be helpful to consider when planning such workshops.

Content of Caregiver Workshops

One significant difference between ACT for recovery workshops for clients and those for caregivers is the discussion points. Caregiver participants tend to want to use the workshops as a forum to discuss or off-load the negative experiences of caring, or both, whereas client participants tended to focus more on their own experiences of psychosis and how to manage these.

As previously mentioned, caring for a loved one with psychosis can be challenging, and caregivers often find it helpful to have a space to discuss their experiences. We find it beneficial for facilitators to meet face-to-face with potential participants prior to starting the workshops. Caregivers who have the opportunity to "tell their caring story" and to off-load before the actual workshops start appear more comfortable in the workshops themselves and do not dominate discussions.

At times we have had to be flexible with the caregiver workshop protocol. We attempt to set the tone of the workshops by explaining, at the beginning, that they are "workshops" in which participants will learn and practice skills. Further, we clarify that we will be asking them to reflect on their experiences with the exercises and how these experiences relate to their caring role. We ask for their permission to interrupt and move on to the next exercise if we feel that the group is moving off topic. Our experience has been that, more often than not, caregivers are receptive to such interruptions, if they are done in a sensitive way. However, it is important to validate the difficult experiences shared by caregivers. One way of ensuring this is to provide a space at the end of workshops, as and when required, to discuss anything that arises in session. However, there are also benefits of going with the flow in some sessions by setting agendas with the whole group and working collaboratively to make decisions about the content of the workshops.

Caregivers of people with psychosis often feel isolated in their roles and may avoid discussing their experiences with people outside their social systems. We have witnessed caregivers share contact details and form strong bonds as a result of attending workshops with people in a similar position. We actively encourage such relationships.

Confidentiality

Often the clients cared for by the caregivers attending the workshops are treated in the same clinical services. One issue that can arise is confidentiality. We make it explicit at the start that the workshops are for people caring for someone experiencing psychosis. To maintain confidentiality, we ask that participants don't provide the full names of the people they care for or refer to them as "son," "partner," "mother," and so forth. Similarly, we also ask that they don't name specific clinical services or mental health professionals, suggesting they instead use "care coordinator" or "doctor."

Identifying Values

As described in chapter 1, a significant component of the workshops is identifying values and what is important. We find that identifying values can be difficult. For example, caregivers occasionally struggle to grasp the concept of values, or they identify goals rather than values. To help clients and caregivers discriminate between goals and values, we sometimes liken them to points on a compass that provide direction in life (Hayes et al., 1999). We often present the following metaphor:

> Our values are like points on a compass. If you were lost and had a compass, you could use it to see if you were, in fact, moving in the direction you wanted to be. For example, suppose you valued moving south. You could use the compass to first make sure that you were facing south, and then pick out a landmark, such as a mountain peak on the southern horizon, to serve as a goal to move toward. As long as you kept the peak in sight, you wouldn't even need the compass itself to know if you were moving in a southerly direction. Now what happens when you actually reach that mountain peak? Are you south? Or is there more south still ahead of you for you to move toward? What if moving south is like being a caring parent (or some other identified

value)? There are many ways to be a caring parent—different goals you could set that move you in that direction—but does it ever end?

Does there ever come a time when you can check being a caring parent off your things-to-do-in-life list, or is it continuous? If that is a central part of what you want your life to be about, can't it continue to be just that as long as you are alive? Even if you outlive all your children, can you still honor that value?

We've also observed that caregivers often highlight values linked to their caring roles. Examples include "I want to be a better caregiver for my son," or "I want to support my partner in a way that helps him comply with his medication." While being careful not to impose our own views on caregiver participants, we highlight that we want them to identify things that are truly important to them. We suggest that through their attendance in the ACT for recovery workshops, they are already connecting with values related to supporting their loved one. We also want to support caregivers as they identify values related to improving their well-being and, thus, to replenishing their reservoirs.

We begin discussions relating to values during the recruitment process and often ask caregivers what they are currently doing that is valuable and important to them. We ask if there is anything else that they want to be doing (goals) but aren't doing at present (starting to identify barriers), as well as why doing this would be important (identifying the values behind the goals).

Another way we overcome issues related to identifying values in larger groups is to discuss examples of common values, with facilitators sharing some of their own values that they are willing to move toward. We have noticed that by repeatedly discussing values in each session, participants' awareness of and connection with their values tend to develop over the course of the sessions. For example, one caregiver repeatedly identified committed actions connected with a specific value (such as applying for a new job), but each week he reported that he had struggled to complete his committed actions (for example, send out a résumé). After several weeks, he reflected that perhaps the goal wasn't so important, but rather he felt that he should be moving toward such values due to external expectations. Facilitators often try to help participants identify what is truly important to them and how they can take steps toward these values.

Further issues arise when caregivers identify conflicts between values. For example, consider a caregiver who identifies the committed action of going for coffee and reading a book to relax. Conflict arises when this person expresses guilt and concern—that by engaging in a value-related committed action (that is, taking time to improve psychological well-being) she is neglecting her role as a caregiver by not being present for the person she cares for. In situations like this, we validate and empathize with such concerns while referring to the reservoir metaphor and asking questions: "By taking a short break to focus on improving your well-being, might this be a way of replenishing your reservoir? What impact might this have on your caring role?" We might also ask, "What does spending time on other valued directions put you in contact with?" We explore how we may be able to use the skills taught in the workshops to help caregivers see these experiences as simply *experiences*.

Video

We use a video of an actor role-playing some of the challenges one encounters when caring for someone experiencing psychosis (available for download at http://www.actforpsychosis.com; see appendix A7 for the transcript). After watching the video, caregiver participants gradually begin to discuss, at their own pace, their own experience of caring. In later sessions, we refer back to the video as a way to reflect on similarities or differences between its content and the workshop participants' caring roles.

Caregivers often relate to the story in this video, and some become emotional while watching it, stating that the video depiction is similar to what they had experienced when their loved one was in a crisis, and that it was painful to recall such memories. We find it helpful to have enough facilitators (for example, two or three) present in the workshops to accompany any participants who wish to temporarily leave the room to compose themselves. At the beginning of the workshops we make it clear that people can leave any time they find workshop content distressing. We explain that a facilitator will check in with them at times to ensure that they know they have the option to leave.

The video is a helpful way of highlighting some of the common complexities that arise when caring for someone with psychosis. However, it may not be applicable to all psychosis caregivers, and we suggest that future facilitators compile vignettes that are applicable to the issues that arise in their specific services.

Consider How Long the Caregiver Has Been in This Role

We offered the ACT for recovery workshops to caregivers of people with established psychosis, and they had all been in caring roles for some time.

Matching caregivers to stage of illness and duration of caring may be useful. We suggest that future facilitators consider how long caregivers have been in the role before opening up a particular workshop to them. For example, caregivers of younger people experiencing early psychosis may be more focused on finding answers, or they may be hopeful that the first episode of psychosis will be the only one (which is possible). They may be less interested in support tailored to the needs of longer-term caregivers, and they may become disheartened after hearing the experience of someone who has been in the caring role for a significant amount of time.

Consider the Nature of the Caring Relationship

Considering the nature of the caring relationship between the caregiver participants and the people they care for can be valuable. We have noticed that parents of people with psychosis have different expectations than those who care for partners. Similarly, adult children who are caregivers tend to have different experiences and issues; they often express more fear and frustration about their role. Discussing such issues with different caregivers prior to starting the workshops can be worthwhile, as it may prepare them for difficult discussions in the workshops.

Follow-Up Groups

The ACT for Recovery study highlights the benefits of a relatively short, four-session protocol for caregiver well-being and psychological flexibility. However, this is not to say that the brief ACT protocol we describe cannot be used as a component of a longer-term support group model. Many of the caregivers who graduated from the ACT for recovery workshops reported that they found the social aspect of meeting other caregivers extremely helpful, and they requested that more sessions be offered. As a result, we have introduced monthly drop-in sessions based loosely on the ACT for recovery protocol. In every drop-in session we review previous committed actions and practice certain noticing and defusion exercises, as requested by the participants. We also provide a space to discuss issues that arise in the caring roles. We have trained several caregivers to take a leadership role in these drop-in sessions, using the training protocol described in chapter 5, with supervision provided by one of the ACT for recovery workshop facilitators. The caregivers in our ACT drop-in sessions have reported that continuing to practice the skills-based components, including noticing and defusion exercises, is extremely helpful, as is the process of making committed actions within a group setting and the continued peer support among participants.

Practical Issues

Due to the nature of the caring role, it is important to consider the timing and location of the ACT for recovery workshops for caregivers. As for timing, we have found it important to offer both daytime and evening workshops, because many caregivers work during the day. We are fortunate to have space that is separate from the one where clients receive routine care. However, this may not be feasible for all service areas, so it is worth considering issues that may arise when caregivers attend workshops at the same place the person they care for is treated.

Occasionally caregivers are unable to attend a workshop due to child care issues or those related to their caring role. When this occurs, we invite them to arrive at the next session early so they can meet with the facilitator and catch up on the content they missed. Our rule of thumb is that caregivers need to attend at least one of the first two workshops of the group protocol, because these involve discussions of the most important aspects of the workshops. If caregivers miss them, we ask that they attend the next set of workshops.

Summary

Caring for people with psychosis involves multiple burdens and challenges, and mental health services increasingly view providing psychological support for caregivers as essential. Caregivers of clients with psychosis have responded positively to the ACT for recovery workshops, and preliminary evidence shows that the well-being and psychological flexibility of participants improved. Our experience also shows that the time commitment of four weekly sessions is acceptable to caregivers, and this brief format allows psychosis services to easily facilitate the sessions. ACT for recovery workshops may therefore be a cost-effective way to provide support and psychological interventions for caregivers to improve their well-being.

As described in chapter 4, the ACT for recovery protocol lends itself to training peer supporters and caregivers to cofacilitate workshops. Caregiver participants who complete the workshops can be invited to cofacilitate and act as "experienced participants," offering their own experiences of using the skills they learned in the workshops and how these skills impacted their caregiving role and well-being.

CHAPTER 3

Adapting ACT Workshops for Acute Inpatient Settings

Written with Rumina Taylor and Georgina Bremner

Our focus in this chapter is to share our experiences of engaging people with psychosis in ACT for recovery workshops in short-admission acute inpatient psychiatric wards. We describe how we have adapted the original intervention so it is briefer and thus can be facilitated on inpatient wards that operate with short and unpredictable admissions.

We know that psychiatric inpatient admissions are costly to both individuals and society, so it is of critical importance to improve the quality of care in order to reduce the number and length of stays. We believe an important step toward raising standards is to increase access to psychological therapies. Group interventions are advantageous, in that they allow participants to share and normalize experiences and they foster a sense of universality. Due to ACT's transdiagnostic approach, we think that it is very fitting for the heterogeneous presentations observed among acute inpatient psychosis populations.

In this chapter we discuss systemic challenges, such as how to engage a particularly distressed group of clients who are not in their usual environment and who have limited access to opportunities, as well as how to work with the wider inpatient staff to promote psychological flexibility and to improve the ward's therapeutic milieu.

Setting the Scene: The Nature of Acute Psychiatric Inpatient Settings

The last fifty years has seen short-admission acute inpatient psychiatric wards undergo a transformation both in the United Kingdom and internationally.

Changing attitudes toward mental health and concerns over living conditions have led to a process of deinstitutionalization. The aim has been to improve these settings and provide better-quality care. Deinstitutionalization has focused on community care and treatment rather than long-stay hospital admissions. The process has occurred at different rates in the United Kingdom (Csipke et al., 2014), Europe (Taylor Salisbury, Killaspy, & King, 2016), and the wider world (Lamb & Bachrach, 2001; Rosen, 2006; Sealy & Whitehead, 2004). Nevertheless, most countries have faced similar challenges as hospital-based mental health care has moved to care in the community. Some critics have argued that this shift has led people with mental health problems to experience greater loneliness, poor physical health (Novella, 2010), homelessness, and inappropriate arrest and incarceration (Lamb & Bachrach, 2001; Rosen, 2006). Deinstitutionalization has been hindered by inadequately funded and difficult-to-access community services (Lamb & Bachrach, 2001), as well as a lack of mental health professionals to provide continuity of care in the community (Taylor Salisbury et al., 2016).

We know inpatient wards continue to provide care and a safe place for those with illnesses that cannot be managed in the community. It is also our experience that ward staff value interactions with patients and would like the opportunity to develop therapeutic and trusting relationships. Indeed, staff report higher satisfaction when they are able to spend time with patients, either for relationship building or therapeutic activities, and through their roles in helping patients recover (Mistry, Levack, & Johnson, 2015). Research also suggests that contemporary nursing care on acute wards can risk a "production line mentality" (Crawford, Gilbert, Gilbert, Gale, & Harvey, 2013, p. 725), with more than half of nursing time taken up by administrative duties, coordination, and managerial tasks, leaving little time for listening, talking, and providing compassionate care to patients (McAndrew, Chambers, Nolan, Thomas, & Watts, 2014).

Ward staff often tell us they lack the time, confidence, skills, and training to work with a difficult-to-engage client group. There may also be a common belief among mental health practitioners that people with serious mental health difficulties who are admitted to the hospital cannot engage in therapeutic relationships (McAndrew et al., 2014). There is now an expectation that interventions be time limited, with prompt discharge to community services (H. Gilbert, 2015), which, in our experience, leads to a focus on medication and stabilization, leaving little time for anything else. Unsurprisingly many patients and their relatives describe acute wards as unsafe and having a negative effect on mental health rather than promoting recovery (Schizophrenia

Commission, 2012). Unfortunately, despite higher staff-to-patient ratios, less time is spent participating in therapeutic activities today than fifty years ago, with a quarter of patients reporting that they have not taken part in formal activities (Csipke et al., 2014). In order to improve acute inpatient care, we believe there needs to be a change, from primarily providing patients with medication and a safe place to using the admission as an opportunity to offer effective treatments (medication, psychological therapies, and social interventions) that promote recovery.

Why Acceptance and Commitment Therapy in Inpatient Settings?

We think that offering psychological interventions on short-admission acute inpatient wards is important to raising the standards, quality, and outcomes of psychiatric inpatient care. However, we know that delivering such interventions can be challenging. The high turnover of patients means interventions need to be relatively short term. We also know that some caregivers view the severity of inpatient psychopathology as problematic for therapeutic engagement. Also, our experience has shown us that patients who are detained may not want to engage and are not necessarily seeking treatment. In order for patients to want to attend interventions provided within an acute inpatient setting, in particular, the interventions need to be interesting, meaningful, and appropriately challenging (Newell, Harries, & Ayers, 2012).

Compared to working in community settings, working with patients on acute wards offers greater opportunities for intervention, as they are more available to spend time with. Of interest to us are group interventions that can provide an important contribution to the ward environment by reducing isolation and providing structure, social support, and access to normalizing and alternative views. We have found groups to be a more efficient use of therapist time, and they can have additional benefits, such as improving the wider therapeutic milieu.

We think that the acceptance and commitment therapy (ACT) approach of enhancing psychological flexibility is especially appropriate for the acute inpatient population. First, by promoting generic psychological skills, it is a transdiagnostic approach (Clarke, Kingston, James, Bolderston, & Remington, 2014), making it fitting for the heterogeneous psychosis presentations observed among inpatient service users.

Second, despite a growing appreciation of the recovery approach, it is our experience that mainstream attitudes continue to view mental health symptoms (particularly psychotic symptoms) as unacceptable. This means that in many mental health settings, recovery continues to be equated to symptom elimination, which can have harmful consequences. We have seen patients unwilling to disclose or share psychotic or other distressing experiences so they could be discharged from the hospital. This reality can mean that individuals in a ward environment may be more likely to avoid or suppress symptoms, leading them to be more fused with their inner world, to become increasingly dominated by their illness, and to retreat from previously valued activities and aspirations (Mitchell & McArthur, 2013). ACT does not focus on eliminating unwanted experiences, and therefore we think it may be more appealing to the patients with long-standing problems who are often admitted for inpatient care. For this population, developing a more accepting stance toward persistent and recurring symptoms (rather than aiming for symptomatic relief) and engaging with more meaningful living are likely to be very beneficial, perhaps more acceptable, processes. We like ACT's focus on specific processes, as it makes brief interventions possible, which is a necessity in short-admission wards.

The South London and Maudsley Inpatient ACT Protocol

In developing our inpatient ACT protocol, we hoped to both improve access to psychological therapies for people within acute care, as well as to add to the limited evidence base. We therefore developed and evaluated the feasibility, acceptability, and potential benefits of an adapted and shorter version of an ACT for recovery workshop within two male acute inpatient wards. The wards were characterized by short-stay admissions, and the majority of the patients experienced psychosis. We describe the adaptations below.

Adaptations for an Inpatient Context

A range of adaptions are needed to ensure that ACT for recovery workshops can be successfully run in inpatient wards. The adaptions include raising the awareness of and familiarity with (both that of ward staff and patients) ACT, encouraging staff to support the workshop intervention, and modifying the format and content of the workshops to better fit the needs of people on the wards and the short admission times.

PROMOTING THE WORKSHOPS TO WARD TEAMS

To prepare for the workshops, we met with the ward teams to provide information about ACT and to ask them to identify suitable participants. We emailed staff a week before and on the morning of the meeting, to remind them about it, and we wrote the meeting time in the ward diary. On the day of the meeting, we visited the ward at the start of the early shift and fifteen minutes before the meeting started to maximize attendance. We kept the meeting as brief as possible (one hour) and tried to make the content of the meeting accessible to the range of staff members attending. We used a slide presentation with information about ACT, its ethos, and its processes, and we facilitated a short mindfulness exercise to provide a taste of what the workshops would be like. We encouraged staff who were keen to cofacilitate workshops to stay behind at the end of the meeting or to email us. While in the meeting we discussed the kinds of patients who could benefit from our ACT workshops and asked staff to identify any potential participants, which we then followed up on. We also attended a weekly multidisciplinary team review in which we discussed all patients and, with our colleagues, identified suitable participants.

In order to maximize workshop attendance and to accommodate the heterogeneous population of inpatient wards, we purposely set broad inclusion criteria and did not make the workshops diagnosis specific. The transdiagnostic nature of ACT is especially appropriate for the setting, meaning participants with different diagnoses and problems can attend. Our goal was for the workshops to provide patients an opportunity to access psychological therapy in an environment that fostered mutual respect between individuals. We encouraged ward colleagues to consider the workshops when developing collaborative care plans with patients, so both patients and staff would see intervention as part of the admission and treatment process.

PROMOTING THE WORKSHOPS TO PATIENTS

We made sure that posters advertising the workshops were displayed on the wards and that leaflets were given to interested and eligible participants. We intentionally promoted workshop attendance as a way to move on from the ward and live a meaningful, fulfilled life, rather than as a way to cope with symptoms or problems. We have found that patients are receptive to this message and are more willing to hear about the workshops when we use it, as many of them have concerns about what to do postdischarge. We met with suitable participants and asked them to complete outcome measures.

We were keen to engage patients who were close to being discharged from the ward, as we felt the workshops, with their focus on recovery and moving forward, could benefit them at this stage—when they may associate leaving inpatient care with feeling stuck in life. We approached this engagement in a way consistent with *transitional discharge*—that is, the time in which inpatient and community services overlap, and inpatient staff continue to work with and support patients after they return to the community. This type of discharge compensates for a sudden loss of relationships the ward provides. There is evidence that transitional discharge reduces readmission rates and improves adherence with appointments and medication (Price, 2007; Reynolds et al., 2004). For these reasons, when participants were discharged before completing the ACT workshops, facilitators invited and actively encouraged (for example, providing telephone reminders and paying for travel to and from the ward) them to attend the remaining sessions.

Due to the pressure on inpatient beds, sudden discharge is common, and it can raise difficult issues for the remaining workshop participants. We tried to encourage participants to return to the ward for the workshops, but we had mixed success. Moreover, the reality of acute inpatient care is that during recovery patient presentations often change. Occasionally participants change and are no longer suitable for the workshops. Examples include when a patient becomes more argumentative, more suspicious of the workshop material, or dominating in discussions—issues that can be disruptive for the other workshop participants. Because ward staff provided handover, we were aware of any potentially difficult presentations before the workshops started. On such occasions, we met with individual patients to see how their week had been and how they were feeling. If we felt it would be difficult for them to participate, we openly communicated this to them as sensitively as possible while holding our values in mind. We offered to meet with individual patients after the workshops to share what was covered and to provide copies of materials. If there were disruptions during the workshops, we reminded participants of the group rules and their values regarding respecting and working with others. We tried to give distressed patients more one-on-one support and asked the ward staff cofacilitating the workshops to do the same. Occasionally we asked nursing staff from the ward to join the workshops and take on a supportive role if required.

On rare occasions, we had to ask participants to leave the workshops, but, again, we did this as sensitively as possible and agreed to meet with them after the workshops to share what was covered.

ADAPTING THE FORMAT OF THE WORKSHOPS

We ran the sessions twice weekly so that the four sessions could be completed within two weeks rather than four (which is the protocol for the community form of ACT for recovery workshops). We did this to accommodate the short admissions of our patients, which are typical of acute psychiatric wards.

Each session had the same structure (described in table 2). We ran closed workshops so the same participants attended each session, enabling rapport and trust to develop. This also made it easier to evaluate the workshops.

There were some systemic challenges to running a closed workshop, especially because most other group workshops on the wards were designed to be open and transdiagnostic, with stand-alone sessions to accommodate the varied nature of admissions and high turnover. Patients who were admitted to the ward after the intervention had started were, unfortunately, unable to access the workshops. On these occasions, we shared information about the workshops with the patients and, if they were interested in attending, placed them on a waiting list. They then started the next set of workshops three weeks later. This worked well, because after three weeks had passed the patients were usually near to discharge and therefore fit with our inclusion criteria.

Running a closed workshop has two major benefits: first, it allows each session to build upon material from the last, and second, it provides a safe and supportive space for participants to develop a sense of connectedness and to share personal experiences. A closed workshop does require some homogeneity in clinical presentation (that is, more disruptive clinical presentations are deemed unsuitable), and it's important to ensure that both ward staff and patients understand this. It was quite disruptive when staff encouraged patients to attend halfway through a session when the patients were not suitable due to their clinical presentation, and it was difficult to explain to some patients why they were not able to attend. If participants were acutely unwell, we tried to manage this by reminding participants of the group rules more regularly and by working with them on a more one-on-one basis, as described above.

We aimed to have four to six participants in each workshop, with two therapists. Each session was only fifty minutes long, to better suit the presentations of acute patients and to compensate for any cognitive difficulties. Most participants, many of whom experienced chronic, distressing, and often treatment-resistant psychosis, were able to tolerate fifty-minute sessions, to engage with the material, and to reflect on personal experiences.

We supported session content by writing key points on a flip chart, by watching the passengers on the bus video (available for download at http://www.actforpsychosis.com), and by assisting participants to complete individual worksheets to record personal values, barriers, goals, and committed action plans, which are included in the original ACT for recovery workshops (see part 2). We provided refreshments and created a relaxed and welcoming atmosphere to further encourage attendance.

We didn't provide follow-up booster sessions, as we deemed this less feasible for the acute environment, in which discharge rates are relatively high. Additionally, our experience has shown us that, after a certain period of time, patients are less keen to return to the ward due to the difficult memories they associate with it.

INVOLVING WARD STAFF IN THE WORKSHOPS

Staff involvement was helpful for identifying suitable participants, and staff encouraged attendance both by reminding patients and by ensuring that other appointments did not coincide with the workshops. Staff cofacilitators tried to ensure that other team members understood that the workshops were closed and who should be attending them. It was helpful to put the names of the patients participating in the workshops in the nursing office and ward diary; doing so helped prevent unsuitable patients from attending. We believe that staff support plays a role in high attendance rates.

Having ward staff involved in the workshops as cofacilitators was helpful, as it promoted the idea of common humanity and reduced the perception of "them" and "us." Working alongside other members of the ward team can reinforce the message that workshop attendance is part of treatment and hospital admission (Radcliffe & Smith, 2007). We therefore extended invitations to ward staff to attend the workshop as either participants or cofacilitators, increasing their sense of ownership of the workshops. Supporting other staff members with individual and group interventions is thought to be particularly pertinent in inpatient settings, where the psychological impact needs to extend to the whole ethos of the institution (McAndrew et al., 2014; Radcliffe & Smith, 2007).

Many nursing and occupational therapy staff members expressed interest in cofacilitating the workshops. Initially staff members attended the workshops as participants, and then we encouraged them to become more involved by cofacilitating the workshops alongside the lead facilitators. After observing and completing the workshops, we provided staff members with information about ACT and its key components. Before each workshop staff cofacilitators met with one of the lead facilitators to plan the session. A debrief and supervision were also provided following each workshop. We created a manual based on the ACT for recovery workshops, which we followed in each session.

Some ward staff were anxious about cofacilitating the workshops. The planning and debriefing sessions were vital, and some staff members noted that having a manual to follow was containing and made cofacilitation possible. Some staff members particularly enjoyed being involved in a group intervention, as it was different from their usual role, encouraged greater therapeutic contact with patients, and taught them skills they could use moving forward in their own practice. Using staff to deliver group interventions via cofacilitation was a useful training model to disseminate expertise and skills in the practice of psychological therapies, which, in turn, could help develop a more therapeutic ward environment.

Although we extended invitations to all staff members, a number of them highlighted difficulties with participating, including being released from their duties; some lacked an interest in exploring psychological groups altogether. A continuing challenge will be integrating ACT principles into the wider ward milieu. This will be especially challenging given that ACT principles, such as nonjudgmental awareness of difficult internal experiences, can contrast with the medical model of symptom control and reduction that continues to dominate inpatient settings. A key component for integrating these principles is continued staff education, both through ward-based teaching sessions and the sharing of psychology skills through modeling and coworking.

ADAPTING THE WORKSHOP SESSION CONTENT

Because individuals engage in less values-based action during crisis (Mitchell & McArthur, 2013), our four-session protocol emphasized participant values more than the ACT for recovery protocol. We also felt that, in a setting where building rapport with patients can be difficult, a focus on recovery goals and values for living would motivate patients to attend the workshops and engage them to a greater extent. Each session was structured around personal values. For example, every session looked at what values are, at what internal and external barriers get in the way of pursuing personal values, and at ideas for working with barriers. And, we asked participants to set values-based goals they could work toward throughout the week. These were revisited in every session.

As set out in the ACT for recovery protocol, the intervention was based principally around the passengers on the bus metaphor, which we discussed every session and illustrated via video, discussion, and role-playing. This metaphor provided a consistent narrative thread and allowed patients to explore issues, such as personal values, committed actions, barriers, thought fusion, and mindfulness. Participants have found it particularly helpful to act out the metaphor within sessions (Johns et al., 2015). Previous research demonstrated the feasibility, acceptability, and value of mindfulness skills for acute inpatients (Jacobsen et al., 2011), and we were therefore keen to include such experiential exercises. As recommended, we chose concrete exercises from the manual, shortened them to five minutes (see table 2), and provided more therapist support through greater verbal instruction and discussion in session.

Each session followed the same format:

1. An exercise to identify values (values card–sorting exercise; Harris, 2014)

2. A barriers-to-values exercise

3. The passengers on the bus metaphor

4. An introduction to mindfulness exercises as a way of being with unwanted experiences so one can pursue values; these exercises promote defusion or acceptance and include the three-minute breathing space, leaves on the stream, noticing others' values, the concept of willingness using the pushing against the folder metaphor, and mindful eating of a slice of cake

5. Discussions of committed action from the previous session

6. Setting between-session committed actions (see table 2)

Participants did find it challenging to set meaningful and relevant committed actions that they could complete between sessions. This seemed to be due to the limited opportunities to pursue certain goals within the acute inpatient setting. For example, a number of patients chose "education" as their value, but they felt the hospital setting restricted what meaningful actions they could commit to that would be in line with this value.

To handle this situation, we encouraged participants to focus on values that better lent themselves to the ward environment (for example, friendship or helpfulness). This "making lemonade when life gives you lemons" approach is about promoting psychological flexibility skills in the ward environment. We think this is an ACT-consistent approach, in that it encourages participants to engage with the situation they are in (acceptance), rather than the one they wish they were in. Of course, we did this in the spirit of active acceptance, rather than resignation, and as a way to practice the skills presented in the workshops.

In supporting participants to make small committed actions, we often talked through a typical day on the ward and tried to identify opportunities when they could act on their values. For example, ward rounds and mealtimes were often useful times to practice expressing one's needs or building friendships with others. Greater creativity on the part of both patients and workshop facilitators is needed when it comes to setting and pursuing committed actions. Unfortunately, after the workshops ended, we were unable to follow up on the committed action plans of individual group members, so we do not know the longer-term outcomes of this work.

Table 2. The content of workshop sessions in ACT for recovery in acute inpatient settings

Session Number	Summary of Content
1.	Start with introductions and ground rules. Introduce the key concepts of values, barriers, and committed action using a flip chart, the values card-sorting exercise (Harris, 2014), the passengers on the bus video, and worksheets. Introduce the concept of mindfulness using the three-minute breathing space. Help participants identify a personal value, and set a corresponding committed action to complete during the week.
2.	Start with introductions and a reminder of ground rules. Revisit the key concepts—values, barriers, and committed action—using the passengers on the bus metaphor. Reduce the mindfulness exercise (leaves on the stream) to five minutes, and use it to illustrate struggles with unwanted psychological phenomena. Help participants identify their barriers, or "passengers," that prevent committed action. Revisit the committed action plan to work with values that better lend themselves to the ward environment (for example, friendship or helpfulness). Support participants as they make small committed actions.

3.	Start with introductions and a reminder of ground rules. Perform the exercise of noticing others' values for five minutes. Introduce the concept of willingness (noticing without engaging) using the pushing against folder exercise (five minutes). Act out the passengers on the bus to practice different ways of responding to one's passengers. Revisit the committed action plans.
4.	Start with introductions and a reminder of ground rules. Practice the mindful eating of a slice of cake exercise for five minutes. Recap the values, goals, internal and external barriers, and committed action plans.

Workshop Outcomes

We facilitated the workshops five times in two male short-admission psychiatric wards, in which the majority of patients experienced psychosis. We recruited 30 participants who attended at least the first session of one of the workshops. Their mean age was 40.4 years, and they had an average contact with mental health services of 6.9 years and an average of 2.6 previous hospital admissions. Just under half (46.7 percent) were classified as black or black British, 43.3 percent as white or white British, and 10 percent as Asian or Asian British, which reflects the local population. The majority of participants (63 percent) were admitted involuntarily; 77 percent had a schizophrenia spectrum diagnosis, 7 percent had a diagnosis of emotionally unstable personality disorder, 7 percent had a diagnosis of nonpsychotic disorder, 3 percent had a dual diagnosis, 3 percent had a diagnosis of mental and behavioral disorder due to alcohol, and 3 percent had a diagnosis of mental health disorder not otherwise specified (World Health Organization, 1993).

We asked participants attending our workshops to complete four outcome measures before the first session and after the final session. Additionally, we administered measures of stress and symptom interference (fusion) before and after each session to measure within-session changes. This measure indicated whether attending one or two sessions, which was often the case with sporadic attendance in the inpatient setting, could be beneficial; in such situations, it may be more informative than pre- and postmeasures (Jacobsen et al., 2011). At the end of the four sessions, participants completed a feedback questionnaire, and staff cofacilitators completed a qualitative interview.

Each session had a median of 5 participants, with earlier sessions having more participants than later sessions, reflecting an attrition rate of 26.7 percent. Each participant completed a mean of 3.3 sessions, in line with similar ACT for psychosis studies (Bach & Hayes, 2002), which reflected an average attendance rate of 83 percent. More importantly, all participants stated that they had enjoyed the workshop and would recommend it. The majority (90 percent) felt they had benefited from the workshop and would like to be involved in a similar group again. Many (74 percent) reported feeling better able to cope with their problems after attending the workshop, with only 30 percent reporting that they found it difficult to discuss problems in the presence of others; however, 79 percent felt they benefited from meeting other group members who had similar difficulties. It appears that the passengers on the bus metaphor and personal values are concepts that most people can relate to, which is in line with other studies (Johns et al., 2015).

The outcomes were encouraging, indicating the potential benefits of running ACT workshops within acute inpatient settings. We assessed within-session changes in stress and symptom interference using stress bubbles (Jacobsen et al., 2011), a visual analogue scale with six bubbles gradually increasing in size, from no stress/interference (score = 0) to very stressed/interfering (score = 5). The significant reductions in both stress and symptom interference within each of the four sessions highlights the benefit of attending even just one session. This is particularly pertinent in the unpredictable ward environment, where many patients will only attend one or two sessions.

Scores across a range of outcomes measures point to improvements in terms of self-efficacy, general psychological distress, mindfulness skills, and valued living. Two of the measures, Clinical Outcomes in Routine Evaluation (CORE–10; Barkham et al., 2013) and the Southampton Mindfulness Questionnaire (SMQ; Chadwick et al., 2008), showed significant changes in scores between baseline and postintervention, indicating that participants reported a significant reduction in general psychological distress and a significant increase in mindful responding. This suggests the workshops were successful in developing those ACT skills that were being targeted. Increased scores on the Valuing Questionnaire (Smout, Davies, Burns, & Christie, 2014) indicated that, although not statistically significant, participants were living slightly more in line with personal values after the workshops. However, this lack of a significant increase might reflect the difficulty, from a clinician's perspective, in helping service users in inpatient settings to set meaningful and relevant committed actions that they can complete between sessions, as described above.

The Experience of Running the Workshops: Cofacilitator Feedback

We analyzed the interviews of staff who had taken cofacilitator roles to identify emerging themes. One theme relates to the practical difficulties involved with setting up and running the workshops, such as finding a room big enough and available at the right time. Another key practical issue relates to the implications of having a high turnover of service users, as highlighted by one cofacilitator:

> Patients tend to move on from the ward quickly, which means that some were discharged during the course of the two-week intervention, and so missed the final sessions.

Another area of difficulty was how to manage unsuitable patients. For instance, participants could present very differently from one session to the next, which could be disruptive for other group members. Another source of disruption involved ward staff who were not aware of the closed format of the workshops, which resulted in patients being sent in long after sessions had started or even if they had not attended previous sessions. The following feedback highlights this difficulty:

> With changing shifts and locum [temporary] staff, it was difficult to ensure that all staff understood the workshop's format, as staff are used to psychology groups being more drop in, drop out.

Besides these various practical issues, another theme was the staff's perception of the workshop's positive impact on patient enjoyment and well-being, including participants appearing more settled and euthymic over the course of the sessions. In relation to this, the staff noted the apparent accessibility of the session content. For instance, many felt the interactive metaphors, video material, and focus on values were relatable and understandable to most service users:

> The ACT principles seemed to be successfully understood by patients, as evidenced by their verbal input and reflections during workshop discussions.

Finally, a number of staff members gave feedback about how their involvement in the ACT workshops impacted their own practice; for example, after cofacilitating, some started to incorporate concepts such as values in their individual work:

We did get feedback from medical staff on the ward that the patients enjoyed the workshop, and we communicated some of the key metaphors (for example, driving your bus, and barriers to doing so) with staff so that they could follow up with some patients and use the same language as a way of communicating with some patients, particularly when they are ruminating about a particular topic or [are] fixed on one subject. So, in this way I think it did make an impact on the therapeutic approach on the ward. Yes, I definitely started to use more of the ACT techniques in my individual work also.

Summary

This chapter provided a current overview of the nature of short-admission acute psychiatric inpatient wards and the importance of delivering psychological therapies in such settings. Implementing these interventions can be challenging, although with the appropriate adaptations it is possible. We found that it is feasible to facilitate an ACT for recovery workshop that patients residing in a hospital deem acceptable and helpful. In this chapter we shared our successes and difficulties. In closing, we emphasize that in our workshops we learned the importance of engaging the wider system on wards, working with inpatient staff to promote psychological flexibility.

CHAPTER 4

Peer-Support Cofacilitators
Working Alongside Clients with Lived Experience of Mental Health Issues

This chapter outlines the case for including people with lived experience of mental health issues as peer-support workshop cofacilitators. We outline some of the background and rationale for doing this and discuss the practical issues involved with ensuring such involvement is both effective and recovery focused. We draw both on our broader experience of involving clients with lived experience in this work and on our direct experience from the ACT for Recovery study (as described in chapter 1).

Background to the Peer-Support Role

Central to an ACT intervention is creating a space within which participants can begin to explore their experience of psychosis and develop the tools to move forward with their lives. Such a journey, which involves exploring alternative perspectives and new ways of living, requires an environment of safety. The emphasis on personal recovery from distressing psychosis has increasingly become an integral part of mental health services, having been driven, to some extent, by those individuals experiencing psychosis.

Historically, the way we've described user involvement has been anchored within narratives of "patients" who are passive recipients of services provided by professionals (Tait & Lester, 2005). However, over the past twenty years, service-user-rights movements, such as Mad Pride, and affiliations, such as the Hearing Voices Network, have flourished as individuals increasingly lobbied to have a collective voice heard by mental health services and mainstream society. Positive recovery stories are now more prominent as individuals such as Eleanor Longden, Rufus May, and Pat Deegan not only publicly offer their personal journey but strongly advocate for the rights of people experiencing distressing psychosis. This has led to more vocal demands for greater choice with regard to treatment options and also meaningful participation in how mental health services are set up and delivered. In addition to this strong political argument, journal reviews suggest that involving the users of services can have a broad, positive impact on outcomes, such as service satisfaction and recovery rates (Oliver, Hayward, McGuiness, & Strauss, 2013; Simpson & House, 2002). There is also developing evidence pointing to the positive benefits of peer-support roles with mental health services in terms of reducing inpatient bed use, improvements in mental health outcomes, and increased self-efficacy and self-management skills (Bates, Kemp, & Isaac, 2008; Crepaz-Keay & Cyhlarova, 2012; Forchuk, Reynolds, Sharkey, Martin, & Jensen, 2007; Lawn, Smith, & Hunter, 2008).

Although negative public attitudes about mental health issues have undoubtedly shifted over recent years, there is still substantial room for improvement. Steven Hayes, one of the founders of acceptance and commitment therapy (ACT), writes:

> Those experiencing psychotic disorders are amongst the most stigmatized people on the planet. They are frequently objectified and dehumanized by society. Their unusual experiences and actions are often objects of ridicule or fear. (Morris, Johns, & Oliver, 2013, p. xx)

Despite changes in attitude, people with psychosis are much more likely to come into contact with mental health and criminal justice services and to be forcibly detained for treatment. As a result, individuals receiving mental health services often have different viewpoints about how these services are structured than do service providers and professionals (Dimsdale, Klerman, & Shershow, 1979; Perkins, 2001). As such, service users can work very hard to develop an identity that is not solely defined by the mental health system. This has resulted in the evolution of terminology that now includes "patient," "client," "consumer," "service user," "expert by experience," and "survivor." The umbrella term "peer supporter" captures many different types of activities, and within a mental health context it refers to people with similar or shared experiences offering others support and assistance (Davidson, Bellamy, Guy, & Miller, 2012; Faulkner & Basset, 2012).

Why Use Peer-Support Cofacilitators?

ACT aims to increase the psychological flexibility skills people have in order to help them choose and commit to meaningful life directions. At their heart, ACT recovery workshops aim to equip people with psychosis to do this.

Alongside increased psychological flexibility and meaningful life directions, recovery principles of hope, empowerment, and partnership are crucial to recovery. The workshops emphasize offering people a menu of potential options that may facilitate their recovery journey. From this perspective, it makes sense to have experts by experience at the center of the work, so participants have the opportunity to come into contact and learn from people who are a little further along in their recovery journey, having negotiated obstacles by employing psychological flexibility skills. Also, involving peer-support cofacilitators can help create a space that recognizes the importance of lived experience and can deemphasize expertise that is aloof, distant, and not subject to common psychological processes in psychosis. The ACT model explicitly recognizes that the processes that contribute to "stuckness" in life are common human experiences that apply across the board. This is encapsulated within the two mountains metaphor (outlined in chapter 1), which describes the client and practitioner as each being on different mountains, facing their own different but common struggles. Simply put, given the context of the therapeutic relationship, the practitioner has a unique perspective on the client's "stuckness," and he or she can usefully bring this perspective into the conversation about the individual's recovery journey.

All of these issues highlight why we felt it necessary to involve peer-support cofacilitators in the ACT for Recovery study. We hoped that their additional perspective would enhance and strengthen the workshops. Feedback from previous workshops had indicated that participants very much appreciated and benefited from the knowledge and experience of those further along their recovery pathway. We wanted to create an atmosphere in which workshop participants felt comfortable sharing their experiences, and we believed that peer-support cofacilitators would promote this. We also felt that there was value in having peers model their lived experience of using the skills and exercises we invited participants to practice, particularly how they could be applied within the context of distressing psychosis.

All the workshops in the ACT for Recovery study included peer-support cofacilitators, all of whom had previous experience with serious mental health conditions, such as psychosis and bipolar disorder, and had used mental health services. We recruited peer supporters through local service user networks, and they all had prior experience working as service user consultants. These consulting roles had included a range of activities, including recruiting staff, service planning, and training. Although most consultants had limited experience delivering psychological interventions, some were skilled trainers and group facilitators.

In the following sections, we outline a number of observations and recommendations from our experience recruiting, training, and working alongside peer-support cofacilitators (Great Britain Department of Health, 2006; Tait & Lester, 2005). We also include some of the feedback we received from individual participants and the peer supporters themselves, highlighting their experiences working with and being cofacilitators.

Observations and Recommendations

To involve peer supporters in a helpful manner, it is important to put in place careful systems and procedures that ensure the peer supporters find their experiences personally useful and that they benefit the overall group process as well. The dual principle of recovery focus and effectiveness is fundamental to this work (Oliver et al., 2013). Having a comprehensive support system in place is crucial to an effective peer-support program; it ensures that peer supporters can complete the required tasks. Below we offer a number of observations and recommendations from our experience.

SELECTION

It is important to select peer supporters who have the skills and experience to undertake the role; therefore, a careful selection process is needed. We recommend carrying out an informal selection process by which the position is advertised through local peer-support mental health networks. It is important to be clear about the nature of the workshops in the advertising, stating that they involve working alongside an experienced cofacilitator and that training and support are provided.

We suggest conducting brief interviews to talk through the requirements of the position and also to assess an applicant's level of experience and comfort with facilitating groups. The interview is an opportunity to ask candidates if they require additional support in order to successfully participate. The interview also offers you the opportunity to discuss the nature of the commitment and to ensure that the candidate is capable of preparing for and attending all the training, supervision, and workshop sessions. It is useful to be clear that you are recruiting peer supporters to be "experts by experience" within the workshops, a role that includes cofacilitation and possibly some disclosure of their lived experience, should they feel comfortable with this.

It is also useful to highlight to candidates that though they will be trained to cofacilitate this particular workshop under supervision, this training does not constitute a formal or actual qualification—meaning they can't go on to offer counseling or therapy services themselves.

PAYMENT

Payment is an important issue; it reflects the valuable contribution that peer supporters offer. In addition, payment implies the expectation that you require high-level participation and involvement. As such, we recommend that, when possible, peer supporters are compensated for their time, including payment for facilitating workshops, attending supervision, and preparing for workshops. Travel expenses should also be covered. Some peer supporters may be receiving government benefits, so you should consider the impact of payment carefully to ensure any earning caps are not exceeded. In such cases, it might be more helpful to have the peer supporter work in a voluntary capacity.

TRAINING

It is likely that peer supporters will need considerable training on the ACT model, the delivery of the manual, and issues related to workshop facilitation. Within the ACT for Recovery study, some peer supporters had prior experience with acceptance and mindfulness practices, whereas others were new to this approach. As such, we developed a one-day training session (discussed further in chapter 5) in which we delivered the workshop program, in part, experientially, running through the key exercises of each session. In the second half of the training, we encouraged peer supporters to facilitate exercises in small groups, and trainers offered feedback. The training sessions had a maximum of ten participants, which allowed the trainers to attend to individual training needs as they arose. The training sessions also included other mental health professionals who would be joining the study, and peer supporters reflected afterward that this mix helped them feel included as part of the wider team.

In the training we also discussed the peer-support cofacilitator role within the workshops, emphasizing that we did not expect peer supporters to lead the workshops, rather they would work alongside an ACT-experienced health professional. We also introduced peer supporters to the training manual and the overall structure of the workshops. We offered practical tips to help them develop the required cofacilitation stance, which was open, supportive, and nonconfrontational. We talked about how to manage difficult situations within the workshops, such as displays of high emotion or arguing. Although these experiences were rare, we wanted to be sure that peer supporters felt able to air concerns and were equipped to manage such situations should they happen.

SUPERVISION

Supervision is an integral part of any peer-support work, and it's particularly necessary for work that is complex and potentially emotionally taxing. We recommend that, in addition to a comprehensive training package, weekly group supervision sessions are provided to all peer supporters for the duration of the program (see chapter 6 for further discussion). In this space, consideration can be given to both content and process issues, including practical advice regarding the facilitation of particular exercises and also time to practice, as necessary.

In the ACT for Recovery study, peer supporters generally acknowledged that, while the role was very interesting, there were elements that were stressful, often related to anxiety associated with the facilitation role or feelings of not being able to engage in the workshop in a competent manner. The supervision groups created a space where such issues could be aired, validated, and normalized.

In addition, it may be necessary to emphasize the importance of peer supporters taking care of themselves and being responsive to their own mental health needs. In order to be responsive to individual needs, it is useful to provide individual supervision sessions to discuss confidential concerns that might arise. Occasionally the mental health issues of some peer supporters impacted their role. When this happened, we worked with the peer supporters to help them determine if they needed help and how to access it. Although these occurrences were rare, we wanted to ensure that the health of peer supporters was a priority.

A key issue addressed in supervision related to the disclosure of mental health experiences. Workshop participants were aware that peer supporters with lived experience of mental health issues would cofacilitate the sessions, but we gave no information beyond that. We encouraged peer supporters to make a personal choice about the amount of personal information they disclosed, considering what felt comfortable to them and what might be helpful for the group. We also encouraged peer supporters to discuss their own experiences of doing the exercises during the workshops (as all facilitators were encouraged to do).

NEED FOR FLEXIBILITY

To help peer supporters facilitate to the best of their abilities, it's important to remain flexible. This can mean offering practical support, such as printing necessary worksheets and manual copies (not all peer supporters will have access to printing facilities). It can also involve reminding peer supporters of supervision meetings or workshop sessions with phone or text messages.

Within workshop sessions, it can be useful to flexibly respond to peer supporters' level of confidence and skill in leading exercises. For example, in a first session they may lead only a brief, less complex exercise (such as a mindful breathing exercise), and the lead facilitator then carries out the post-exercise inquiry, modeling the stance and responses. As confidence grows, peer supporters can take on more complex components. When possible, it's useful for peer supporters to be involved in more than one workshop, so they can build their skills in subsequent workshops.

Feedback on the Peer-Support Role

Overall, involving peer supporters in the intervention added to the complexity of the ACT for Recovery study, both in terms of additional recruitment and supervision processes. However, it undoubtedly added to the richness and effectiveness of what we offered. Most importantly, including peer supporters helped increase the validity of the model for participants. Hearing from someone with lived experience of mental health issues who had also used the ACT model personally helped participants feel comfortable more quickly within the workshops, as noted by a participant in a poststudy interview:

> I think it was useful that a person who has gone through the experience of having a mental illness wants to share their thoughts and feelings… The comments showed that they had similar experiences, which improved their credibility. I felt I could open up more.

This comment reflects that the presence of peer supporters helped participants recognize the universality of experiences, such as distress. It is perhaps this factor that made participants more willing to open up and approach distress in new and more helpful ways. Broadly, the presence of peer supporters strengthened the bonds of collaboration and partnership in the workshops. This is critical for the ACT model, which seeks to reduce the struggle with experiences that are stigmatizing or exclusionary. The comment above also speaks to the point that participants felt safer within the workshop, which was especially important, as the brevity of the intervention didn't offer participants a lot of time to develop relationships.

Participants also spoke about how having peer supporters overtly modeling the skills described and taught in the workshops gave them a realistic appreciation of how to apply these skills. This has more impact than does modeling from professionals, whom participants tend to view as less authoritative because many have not had direct personal experience with serious mental health issues and psychosis. As a result of having peer supporters acting as ambassadors for recovery, participants described feeling very hopeful for their own recovery journey.

Within the workshops for caregivers, participants also reported that the peer supporters were extremely helpful and beneficial. Caregiver participants described feeling hopeful that positive changes could be made, and that they and their loved ones were on a similar journey, as one noted:

> I found it useful. It gave me hope that people's lives can be changed… That we were all going through it together.

There were also clear benefits for the peer supporters themselves. Interviews performed after the workshops were completed indicated two main themes of benefit. First, in the role of cofacilitator, peer supporters viewed themselves as equals with other mental health professionals. This was an important experience for many peer supporters, in that it helped reduce the sense of stigma and self-stigma associated with mental health issues. The following sentiments of two peer supporters illustrate this point:

> My self-image has changed… I see myself differently. Some of the stigma that I experienced, which I internalized, is no longer impacting on me the way it was before.

> It was probably the first time I felt a proper equal to the professionals, which is, you know, not a bad thing.

Peer supporters also felt it was useful to hear some of the self-disclosures of their professional cofacilitators (see chapter 5). As noted by two participants, this further reinforced the notion of equality among cofacilitators:

> I remember, looking at the other therapists and being sort of surprised that other people had issues that—you know, there's kind of the assumption all the time that therapists and people in this industry, sort of, they're perfectly fine and they don't have any hang-ups, and that [professional cofacilitator self-disclosure] was a real eye-opener and actually very helpful to see.

> I found it actually quite interesting, to see how the therapists I worked with were willing to make themselves vulnerable. They were willing to allow themselves into it, which is very uncommon in conventional therapeutic space.

Another theme that emerged was that the cofacilitator role clearly helped peer supporters progress with their own recovery journey. A number of them spoke about the benefits of learning through teaching others, and how this subsequently had a positive personal impact. It was important that the cofacilitator role both enhanced the intervention and was recovery focused for the peer supporters themselves. One peer supporter noted this process:

> It [peer-support role] also allowed me to tackle stuff that in the past I left to one side, emotional stuff, which I would never have been able to start to confront.

A Peer-Support Personal Account

To illustrate the experience of cofacilitating the ACT for recovery workshops from a personal perspective, we asked one of the peer-support cofacilitators to reflect on the experience.

> My involvement in the ACT for Recovery study has allowed me to continue on a journey of self-discovery. It has allowed me to defuse from the negative narratives often associated with the limitations of service user involvement. In turn my self-image (self-as-context) began to change. I began reconnecting with the core values that have guided my actions and informed my beliefs. Reconnecting with my values empowered me to take committed action fueled by my values, confirming and affirming my self-as-context. I have also been willing to embrace the psychological barriers (passengers) that function both internally and were influenced by external cues and the social contextual variables within which they occurred. The result has been to enable me to achieve goals which until very recently have felt too difficult and not worth taking on.
>
> I have digested the Hexaflex model in an academic, intellectual, philosophical, and experiential fashion. I accepted the distressing emotions and tried not [to] judge them or be driven by them. In the past I have often run away from the cause of the distressing emotions (experiential avoidance). There were occasions during workshop supervision where I vented my anger and frustration, but chose not to act on them. I allowed myself to continue in my value-guided direction and felt motivated to keep following this. I'm now writing this reflection and am about to start voluntary work within a psychology service. I would

not have made progress toward my value-guided goals if I had not been willing to let go. I still face considerable challenges as I am unemployed and on government benefits. I now see this as an opportunity, more than a struggle or burden. Actively looking for employment involved approaching a psychology service to explore the possibility of volunteering and involved meeting the volunteer coordinator in the outpatient building where I had been treated. I believe this has been a powerful affirmation of my recovery journey and a clear example of self-as-context.

My journey of recovery has been a long and difficult one; cofacilitating the ACT for recovery workshops has allowed me to continue on that journey. I began with a simple question: Why am I interested in mental health? The simple answer is "know thyself," a journey which began with an examination of classical philosophy and led to me completing a psychology degree. The greatest obstacle I encountered on my recovery journey has been hope; I came to accept hope via acknowledging my despair. In ACT terms, I recognized my "passengers" and came to accept and to some extent love them and allowed them to stay on the bus!

Summary

Including peer supporters in the ACT for Recovery study was one of the key ingredients to its success. We wholeheartedly encourage you to find a way to include the peer-support perspective in your work of bringing ACT ideas and interventions to people experiencing distressing psychosis. This is not always a straightforward process, and how you do it will depend, in part, on your service setting and the systems in place for coproduction efforts. Including peer supporters is likely to complicate the setup and delivery of ACT for recovery workshops, and doing so will require additional time for supervision and support. However, our experience taught us that adding peer supporters adds a flavor of richness to the intervention.

Being of a pragmatic mind-set, we suggest that you start small with how you involve peer supporters in your intervention. Small steps could include seeking detailed feedback after each session or consulting with people who already completed the workshops to find out how the sessions could be improved. Another option is to invite participants back to future workshops to act as experienced participants who take part but also benefit new group members with their previous experience. All of these methods can tap into the wealth of knowledge and experience that peer supporters have to offer to the workshops.

Finally, it is important to remember the dual principles of effectiveness and recovery focus within peer-support work. The work should both make a meaningful contribution to the workshops while keeping the recovery needs of peer supporters paramount. The suggestions we made here go some way to ensuring these standards are met.

CHAPTER 5

Running Successful and Effective Workshops

Training

In this chapter, we will describe several aspects of running successful and effective ACT for recovery workshops. Our focus is on how to develop the support needed to ensure that the workshops are led in ways that are consistent with the ACT model and adhere to the protocol described in this book.

The ideas and advice about leading groups that we present are relevant to anyone who is developing skills to run ACT workshops. We also outline and give tips on how to train facilitators to run the workshops in ways that are engaging, are ACT consistent, and promote the open, aware, and active skills that support personal recovery. In addition, we describe how to train people with lived experience to be cofacilitators in the workshops.

Training

We appreciate that readers of this manual come to acceptance and commitment therapy from various backgrounds. For some, the ACT model is very familiar, and their interest may lie in how the approach is modified for the needs of people recovering from psychosis. Others may have limited knowledge about the ACT model and how the skills of psychological flexibility are taught and promoted in a group setting. Some readers will be very familiar with running groups, whereas for others this is a new experience!

To create a group experience that promotes ACT skills, we have found that it is crucial to take the time to train workshop therapists. Just as a sports team benefits from practicing before a game, so to do cofacilitators who prepare and find the best ways to cooperate before running workshops using ACT. In the following sections, we describe how you can create a training environment that supports workshop facilitators so they can do ACT well.

Our Experiences Training Workshop Facilitators

The ACT for Recovery study is the product of years of development. Joseph Oliver and Eric Morris (two of the authors) started running workshops in an early intervention service for psychosis several years before the ACT for Life and ACT for Recovery studies were conducted to evaluate the efficacy of the workshops. With the early intervention service, our intention was to create engaging and fun workshops for the young people accessing it, many of whom had histories of low educational achievement and a distrust of authority figures. These young people helped teach us how to do ACT in a way that wasn't… well, *really lame*—that is, the type of intervention in which a teacher-type figure spends lots of time telling participants what they need to learn, or in which there is an implicit message that the participants are the problem. For the young people we worked with, not offering lame workshops was especially important, particularly on days when they had lots of intrusive thoughts or voices, or it had taken all of their willpower just to make it to the workshop.

This experience helped us to learn how to run ACT workshops *with all the edges worn off*. What we mean by this is that due to having to sustain the interest of young people with distressing psychosis, we had to come up with a fun, accessible, and jargon-free way to introduce the ACT model. It also meant that we needed to find ways to make the psychological model more active—such as having metaphors come alive by acting them out, using pictures and illustrations, and having briefer, focused mindfulness and noticing exercises. These same considerations were important when we initiated a trial of the workshops for people who had been accessing mental health services for a long period of time (such as those engaged in recovery services and social-inclusion initiatives). This more active and down-to-earth way of presenting the ACT model appeared to resonate with many of these participants, too.

While we agreed on how the workshops should be run, and had shared the experience of doing the workshops in the early intervention service, when it came to teaching people how to run the workshops we discovered that it was a challenge to transmit these ideas. It was also clear that, when working with other mental health professionals in our service, we were the most familiar with the ACT model, and though our colleagues had experience with mindfulness practices, they found combining this skill with other elements of ACT challenging. It was a challenge for us to think of how to train other people.

We had to think of ways to teach our colleagues how to run the workshops without expecting that they would devote as much time to learning ACT as we had! (Otherwise, we were going to have a problem with being able to share the workshop protocol and to do it at a scale that would be useful to our mental health services). We did find ways to do this, which enabled us to conduct the ACT for Life study (described in chapter 1), with other health professionals cofacilitating the workshops with us.

For the ACT for Recovery study, we were faced with a new challenge: How would we help experts by experience** (peer-support facilitators) learn the ACT model and protocol? These people with lived experience had not run therapeutic groups before. An additional challenge for us was that we wanted peer-support facilitators to be able to use their expertise from their own personal recovery journeys to enhance the workshop experience. So, we did not want them to become solely ACT-workshop therapists. Our intention was that the peer-support facilitators would bring the *authenticity* of lived experience and add *credibility* about personal recovery. We hoped that they would find links with ACT, which we believed was a recovery-consistent model.

Promoting Recovery-Oriented Practice Through ACT Workshops

In the following sections we describe how we train workshop facilitators in general, and then we discuss how we teach additional skills to peer-support facilitators who may not have had training in running therapeutic groups. We also consider the support and supervision needs of peer-support facilitators (some of which are discussed in chapter 4) while they prepare and lead workshops.

As described in chapter 1, we believe that ACT provides an evidence-based technology for doing therapy consistent with recovery principles. Supporting personal recovery involves interacting with workshop participants in ways that strengthen an open, aware, and active approach to pursuing a life of purpose and meaning. This means supporting the *process* of personal recovery: different people make different choices about what matters to them.

For clinicians who are less familiar with recovery principles, the experience of using the ACT model—and its applicability to their own lives—is one way to gain a sense of how personal recovery works. By using the ACT model, they will get a sense of the universality of pursuing personal meaning and purpose,

---

** We recognize that health professionals can, of course, also be experts by experience. Several of our colleagues are people who have experienced serious mental illness and bring this perspective into their clinical work. In this chapter we use the "experts by experience" and "peer-support facilitator" descriptors to refer to workshop facilitators acting as peers to the group participants, rather than performing the primary role of a health professional. Some health professionals leading the ACT workshops may also present from the perspective of having lived experience.

which expands one's understanding of ACT, from being simply a treatment model to an approach for achieving well-being and flourishing.

Training Mental Health Professionals as Facilitators

How does one prepare mental health professionals to run ACT for recovery workshops? In our UK National Health Service setting, we have had a variety of professionals facilitate workshops, including psychologists, occupational therapists, social workers, and mental health nurses. When the protocol has been used in other countries, psychiatrists and ward staff in inpatient units led the workshops.

Being introduced to the ACT model can sometimes be challenging for mental health professionals, particularly for those who have not been exposed to it before. This is because ACT sits outside of the disorder-oriented model of health and functioning. Though the medical model of mental health care is frequently criticized as being reductive, in practice many health professionals still work with reductive ideas of disorder, assuming that clients are broken or flawed in some way. Working in a truly recovery-consistent way, in which there is a holistic view of people and a respect for their choices and pursuit of personal meaning, can be a different experience for many health professionals. The ACT-model focus on fostering greater life meaning and purpose through values-based actions can be different for some people, especially when compared to a common mental health focus of seeking to eliminate or limit the impact of symptoms.

Thus, one challenge can be to encourage mental health professionals to respond in a way that promotes active acceptance of experiences, rather than seeking ways to alleviate them. We are not suggesting that people approach mental health problems with resignation (if there is a pragmatic way that will help someone be less distressed and/or disabled over the long term, then this should be suggested). However, we have observed that the general stance of reducing participants' symptoms, with an associated focus on minimizing arousal or negative feelings, can compromise the promotion of personal recovery. Personal recovery may involve positive risk-taking, turning toward feelings of vulnerability, and doing things that may evoke distress to pursue personal meaning. As such, this stance of limiting client distress in a rigid way (costing life purpose and meaning) is less likely to be workable.

When training mental health professionals in the ACT approach, we promote a set of assumptions about the workshop participants:

- It is possible for the participant to pursue a life of purpose and meaning, with the opportunities and situations that are currently available.

- The skills of being open, aware, and active are already in the participants' repertoire (perhaps underused or not applied widely enough).

- There is a lot to learn about how personal recovery is pursued from the participants' lived experience.

- The workshops are about creating experiences for the participants to experiment with using the open, aware, and active skills.

Consistent with the ACT model, the workshops are not built on the assumption that people are "broken" or "damaged." Similarly, while the workshop participants may have diagnoses of serious mental illness, there is nothing in the approach that is based on the idea that the workshops are about fixing something that is "wrong" with them. (In fact, as can be seen from chapter 2, we use the same group format to engage caregivers and others in the ACT workshops.) Again, if the mental health professionals have operated within a framework of considering participants to be disordered in some way, or that the professional should be seen as an expert, this set of assumptions can be challenging for some. (A detailed argument for the limitations of the disorder-oriented approach for psychological and social treatments to recovery is beyond the scope of this manual. We recommend checking out sources such as Richard Bentall's *Madness Explained*, 2004, or the British Psychological Society's report *Understanding Psychosis and Schizophrenia*, 2014.)

Training People with Lived Experience to Be Cofacilitators

In many ways it may be easier to train peer-support facilitators: they may be much more familiar with personal recovery, perhaps having lived experience of doing it. However, there are also challenges: peer-support facilitators will not necessarily come with the degree of mental health knowledge that health professionals have, perform a different role than health professionals, may not be socialized in a professional way of acting, and may have occasions when their own mental health affects their performance facilitating workshops.

We recommend that if you engage peers as partners, consider the issues discussed in chapter 4. Below we will also further discuss supervising peer-support facilitators. We recommend training mental health professionals and peers supporters together. This allows for useful learning for both, and it fosters the universality that is central to the ACT model. In our experience, there have been very powerful and useful moments in training peers and mental health professionals together: both discover the common experiences they share, and there are opportunities to see how the ACT model can help different people. For example, during one of our facilitator training sessions, following several noticing and values exercises, a peer supporter described the moment as the first time in her twenty years of contact with mental health services that she had felt "equal" to professionals. She reflected that this had come about as she witnessed health professionals disclose their own experiences of struggling and vulnerability.

A Training Program for Workshop Cofacilitators

Now we can describe an approach to training facilitators. Typically, we try to offer facilitators at least a full day's training, but preferably two, that we then support with ongoing supervision. Our experience has shown that facilitators need more than a brief training to develop the familiarity and basic skills for running the workshops. It is best to consider how you will support the facilitators as they prepare to run the workshops, while they deliver group sessions, and after the workshops have ended (as you may plan for future group programs). The training sessions have the following goals:

1. Introduce facilitators to the workshops and review session content.

2. Introduce noticing
   - Lead mindfulness and/or noticing exercises.
   - Lead mindful inquiry.
   - Use self-disclosure during mindful inquiry.
   - Determine if workshop facilitators need to have a mindfulness-based practice.
   - Encourage the self-practice of noticing exercises.

3. Introduce ideas about barriers (passengers) and acting on values.

4. Link acting on values with noticing and willingness.

5. Practice defusion exercises.

6. Get in contact with values as directions and commit to action.

7. Provide an opportunity to practice exercises and give general guidance.

INTRODUCE FACILITATORS TO THE WORKSHOPS AND REVIEW SESSION CONTENT

We give each facilitator a copy of the workshop protocol and orient them to an outline of how each session is structured (see part 2). We present the general introduction to the workshops with the rationale that they are about supporting personal recovery. This goal may be different from other mental health interventions, which often focus on symptom reduction, stabilization, or increased functioning (without it necessarily being tied to values-based actions).

We describe the ACT model as a set of psychological flexibility skills that increases people's ability to engage in actions that matter to them and to have lives driven by a sense of purpose and meaning. We present the model as fostering personal recovery through these skills. There are, of course, a myriad of ways that people can pursue their personal recovery—we don't suggest that ACT skills are the only way (a point that is repeated in the workshops; we present the skills so they can be used alongside what participants have already found useful).

We then outline the general structure of each session:

1. Practice mindfulness and/or noticing exercises.

2. Review committed action activities (values-based actions and practicing noticing) for outside of sessions.

3. Review, discuss, and act out the passengers on the bus metaphor.

4. Construct and clarify values and make plans for committed action (in smaller groups).

If the workshops follow this general structure, and facilitators ensure that these elements occur in each session, then there is a good chance that psychological flexibility will be strengthened for participants. It is useful for facilitators to know this, particularly for those workshops sessions when participant sharing and conversation overtake the structure!

INTRODUCE NOTICING

In the training session, we generally introduce *noticing* as a broader set of skills (that includes mindfulness) and as a way of being open and aware, which will foster being active—that is, taking values-based actions.

We have found that there are two important components in teaching mindfulness as a therapeutic skill. First, there is the skill of leading mindfulness exercises, and second, there is the skill of mindful inquiry and talking about mindfulness in a way that shapes this behavior in the workshops.

Lead mindfulness and noticing exercises. The first part of becoming fluent at leading mindfulness exercises is learning how to model them, including such aspects as pacing, tone of voice, and ad-libbing around what participants are instructed to notice. During training facilitators usually start developing fluency by reading the exercise scripts. Typically, they read the scripts too quickly, so that the pacing is off in terms of participants having enough time between instructions to practice noticing, and to then get caught up by experience, and to then find a way back to the exercise "anchor" (or at least the facilitator's voice). Also, reading a script has a different quality than guiding people through an exercise—that is, it can sound like a classroom book reading, rather than words that are said "for effect" or to foster the experience of noticing.

To help facilitators develop their skills for leading a mindfulness exercise, we encourage them to record themselves leading an exercise, and then to try to follow the exercise while listening to the recording. This usually provides useful feedback on pacing and tone (although most facilitators also find that they have to practice willingness toward the experience of listening to their own voice). We also encourage people to develop their own style, so that they can eventually freestyle an exercise without a script.

In leading exercises, there are several points for the facilitators to remember:

- We are promoting all sorts of noticing in the workshops, so facilitators should encourage anything that the participants describe that indicates they are increasing their noticing and awareness. There is no right or wrong way to do noticing; we aren't trying to promote a relaxed state or to develop participants into "mindfulness gurus."

- The aim is not to try to change our experiences: we are simply allowing ourselves to be in a world that seems to be all about doing. So, we encourage participants to let their experiences be just as they are and for them to be just as they are as people.

- We are trying to strengthen the active nonjudgment of experiences. This means observing experiences with a gentle curiosity, kindness, and compassion. We may encourage participants to "just notice" what is happening in their bodies and minds; or we might encourage them to experiment with simply learning to observe their experiences. As best as the participants can, we want to encourage them to open up and allow their experiences to be there, and to just notice them.

- Mindfulness is about noticing the activity of minds and practicing coming back to the present moment.

Lead mindful inquiry. The second part of learning to lead noticing and mindfulness exercises is how to engage workshop participants in mindful inquiry. This inquiry, done after every noticing exercise, reflects the stance we take in the ACT for recovery workshops: each conversation can serve the purpose of promoting psychological flexibility skills.

During the training sessions, we demonstrate how to lead a mindful inquiry using questions, which help participants reflect on the exercise and share experiences by describing them, and this format allows facilitators to shape open and aware responding. The facilitator asks questions, like "What did you notice during the exercise?" and "What experiences did you have?"

The aim is to encourage participants to describe the experiences that arose during the exercise. This way of speaking is progressively shaped over the workshop program, so that descriptions become more present focused over time, with a quality of observation, curiosity, and openness to experience (that is, more open and aware).

When participants first share, you should expect their reflections to be a mixture of descriptions of experiences, judgments, and ways that they struggle or become entangled with what they notice. These are great opportunities for facilitators to help participants distinguish between getting caught up with an experience and noticing it.

So, when participants first share experiences, the facilitator's job is to reinforce anything that participants noticed. This includes seemingly problematic or unwanted experiences with which participants may have struggled. Basically, facilitators want to encourage the group to recognize that, whatever the experience and however entangling it may have been, there was some type of noticing happening. Facilitators can do this with phrases like these:

So you *noticed* that it was hard to concentrate on the exercise?

You *observed* that there was a voice commenting on everything you were doing in the exercise?

You were *aware* that you were getting caught up by negative thoughts while we were doing the exercise?

You experienced relaxation—great *noticing*! Where in your body did you experience this? Did anyone else experience anything similar or different?

Essentially, the facilitator is conveying the message that there is no way to fail a noticing exercise: whatever participants notice, that is their experience, and, with practice, they may be able to observe their experience with curiosity and openness.

We encourage facilitators to offer the opportunity for lots of feedback before responding in detail to any one participant. The most important action is to draw on the group's experience and process, encouraging a social environment in which sharing what participants notice and how they respond is valued.

If a participant shares noticing that is ACT consistent, such as describing the experience, sharing what may get sticky or entangling about that experience, expressing willingness to have the experience as part of a valued direction, or taking a compassionate stance toward herself or the experience, the facilitator should reinforce these reflections and ask further questions about the participant's observing. If participant feedback is not ACT consistent, the facilitator should just acknowledge it and then put the task of observing back to the group by asking participants to share other experiences that they noticed.

It can be tricky when participants report that they found the exercise relaxing. It is important to respond in a way that reinforces the noticing behavior, while not suggesting that relaxation is the primary aim. If this arises, we suggest emphasizing that this is what the participant noticed on this occasion. Highlight that relaxation can be a bonus of doing the exercises, but that the main aim is noticing. This is an important point for facilitators to grasp in training: while workshop participants may have calming experiences, it is important that facilitators reinforce the *noticing* rather than chasing the feeling of relaxation. When running the workshops, we usually respond by drawing attention to the observation that the participant noticed relaxation on this occasion, but that not all noticing produces positive experiences. This is an important point for participants to understand for future exercises; it helps them learn that negative experiences that arise from noticing exercises are not a sign of failure or of something being wrong.

After a participant has shared an experience, and the facilitator has encouraged reflection, we then prime further sharing. Typically we invite other group members to describe their experiences in noticing by asking, "What else did you notice? The same as other people or something different perhaps?"

Use self-disclosure during mindful inquiry. When no participants share experiences (which can happen during the first couple of noticing exercises), we encourage facilitators to share their own experiences. This has the intended purpose of modeling the type of sharing that we are encouraging in the workshop. The types of self-disclosure involved in ACT may be unfamiliar to facilitators (Westrup, 2014). The principle in the workshops is to share experiences that arise while noticing, which enables participants to discover that everyone has experiences with which they struggle or get caught up in. In addition, in seeing how the workshop facilitators respond to each other, such self-disclosure may set the scene so that participants are more willing to share their experiences.

Following the excellent advice from Westrup (2014), we encourage facilitators to consider the purpose of their self-disclosure: Is it likely that it will promote psychological flexibility for the participants in some way? Will the sharing positively impact the group process? Are you saying something in order to feel like you're contributing, being clever, trying to explain ACT, or for some other reason? We have found that, over the course of the workshop sessions, facilitators need to offer less self-disclosure to promote general group sharing, because participants start to open up more about their experiences and struggles.

Finally, it is important to remind facilitators of a (lightly held) rule: when you are talking about ACT, you aren't doing ACT. The mindful inquiry should focus on workshop participants observing experiences, with brief reinforcing of willingness and observing, rather than lead into long discussions about the merits of ACT. We want to limit trying to convince participants that noticing is "the way" to recover. The workshop is more about fostering curiosity and openness to experience and exploring and constructing valued directions than fixing people.

Determine if workshop facilitators need to have a mindfulness-based practice.

Yes, we think that to be able to teach the skills in the workshops, facilitators need to have practiced mindfulness for a sustained period. Talking about mindfulness is not the same as *doing it*. Being able to describe how mindfulness can allow an openness to experiences, and to shape this in others, does involve a personal familiarity with the practice.

One way to do this is to practice and reflect on the very mindfulness and noticing exercises they will lead in the workshops. In the training sessions, there is opportunity to practice mindfulness exercises with other facilitators and to get feedback about how to lead exercises and do the inquiry that follows. We suggest that this is a minimum to be able to facilitate the workshops with skill. To develop a strong and fluent familiarity with mindfulness, we recommend that facilitators engage in a period of practice and study. For example, facilitators could participate in a mindfulness course that involves regular meetings (such as an introduction to mindfulness course that meets over an eight-week period), and then engage in self-practice for a period of six months, whether that be through personal practice using audio recordings or online apps or meeting with a group that practices mindfulness, or all of the above.

We recommend this familiarity through self-practice, because in the workshop facilitators will engage participants in an experiential way of learning how to use mindfulness to strengthen values-based action. Also, facilitators will also develop a good sense of what it is like to sustain a daily practice of present-moment awareness and observing experiences. Having familiarity will also be helpful when facilitators support participants as they bring these skills into their daily lives.

We also recommend that facilitators become familiar with mindfulness consistent with the ACT model—that is, learning mindfulness in a flexible way by trying a variety of exercises and bringing a mindful approach to everyday life. Cultivating a practice of mindfulness that strengthens the facilitator's values-based actions is even better. Key to the ACT approach to mindfulness is using present-moment awareness, defusion, acceptance, and perspective-taking as skills that empower participants to act in valued directions. We suggest that facilitators link their mindfulness practice with acting on their personal values. This again will provide the experiential knowledge that can inform skilled responding during the workshops.

Encourage the self-practice of noticing exercises. In the ACT for Recovery study, we encouraged participants to practice noticing and mindfulness exercises outside of sessions. We typically gave participants recordings of noticing exercises on a compact disc, on a USB stick, or via an online link.

A regular item on the committed action activities list is practicing noticing exercises. While a number of participants do practice these exercises at least a couple of times, it is typical for them to gain the majority of their noticing experience in the workshop. However, it is still important to provide participants with the tools to learn from their own experience, and the recorded exercises are useful for this.

While there are noticing exercises that you can download (see http://www.actforpsychosis.com), we think it is better if you record your own exercises to use in your workshops. Not only will they be in your own voice, which will be familiar to the participants, doing so also provides useful experience in leading noticing exercises.

INTRODUCE IDEAS ABOUT BARRIERS (PASSENGERS) AND ACTING ON VALUES

A set piece in the training is to present the passengers on the bus metaphor in the various forms used in the workshops. This metaphor is *the* central exercise in the workshops, and as often as possible facilitators should try to link back to this metaphor. Passengers on the bus is used as a *scaffolding* metaphor, from which facilitators hang various bits of workshop content. It provides a consistent, central story for participants.

In the training sessions facilitators should discuss the various barriers that we as humans can experience. These include both internal barriers ("passengers," or thoughts, memories, feelings, sensations, and urges) and external barriers (practical issues such as having opportunity, money, time, resources, other people, and so forth). Facilitators should be clear that we are interested in helping participants find different and helpful ways to respond to their passengers, so that they can make the most of the situations they are in and act on their values. It is useful to notice that people may have more ability to respond differently to internal barriers than external ones.

We encourage facilitators to be sensitive to the challenging lives that participants with serious mental illness can have. We are not presenting values-based actions as a panacea or unrealistically optimistic approach to common challenging situations, such as family discord, substandard housing, or limited finances, that people disabled with mental illness can face. The ACT for recovery approach is not one that suggests to participants that life could be better if they just did more… It may be that by connecting with chosen life directions, some participants find that there is need to change routines or relationships or, indeed, to be doing fewer things that they find draining. (For caregivers who participated in the workshops, this latter point has proven to be an important one.)

LINK ACTING ON VALUES WITH NOTICING AND WILLINGNESS

Values-based actions are both supported by the skills of noticing and willingness and become a focus for these skills. We try to impress upon facilitators that the ACT skills are interrelated. Thus, by encouraging a stance of willingness, the questions become "Willingness to experience what?" and "Willingness for what purpose?" We are only encouraging participants to try out willingness in order to enhance their ability to act on values, not because the group or the facilitators expect it.

People often have the stereotype that individuals who are really skilled in mindfulness spend all day in a Zen-like state, unattached to the concerns and worries that the rest of us have. The ACT approach to mindfulness is not to chase a state like that (if it is even possible). We kind of joke that people who live like that, detached from the world, live in caves or shrines and focus on their spiritual growth. Instead, the type of mindfulness we are trying to develop in workshop participants is more for the villagers who live down in the valley away from the caves and shrines. People like most of us, who have responsibilities and concerns, loved ones, bills to pay, and everyday lives. The ACT approach to mindfulness is certainly to encourage an open, aware, and active approach to daily life. This means that for most of us, we may have mindful moments, but we may find it hard to sustain a daily mindfulness practice. And that's okay. We think ACT is about strengthening these skills so that they are more available as an option during daily life. Values-based actions and choices, as part of personal recovery, can frequently involve moments of contact with vulnerability, discomfort, and unwanted experiences. The mindfulness skills of noticing, openness, nonjudgment, and acceptance that we promote in ACT can strengthen participants' ability to cope with these experiences, enabling them to do the things they care about. Being in the moment and doing what you care about, is the messy business of living a full and rich life.

This touches on an important point: the focus of ACT for recovery is to *add to* the coping skills that the workshop participants already have. We know that participants have already developed ways to cope with their experiences and histories, and we work to acknowledge and honor this in the workshops. Certainly, the stance we take as workshop facilitators is to validate that even getting to the workshop some days may involve using coping skills to just manage the moment. In fact, coming to the workshop may be a committed action in its own right.

The ACT for recovery approach is to present the open, aware, and active skills as *additional ways* to enable the moment to be about values-based action.

The style of the group conversation is not to suggest that people are coping in poor ways, or to indicate that the ACT skills are better in some way. Because we are interested in encouraging workshop participants to learn from their experience, we present the idea of values-based behavior as consistent with personal recovery, and we encourage experimentation with noticing and acceptance skills (mindfulness). We are *genuinely interested* in the experience of the participants who are practicing the mindfulness exercises, many of whom are doing so for the first time. Because we have adapted the mindfulness exercises so they are more engaging for people recovering from psychosis, and we have good evidence that these exercises are safe and acceptable (Chadwick et al., 2016), we can focus on whether introducing them in the group experience is engaging for the participants. Most participants have described some benefit from engaging in the workshop exercises, even as a shared experience, and even if some participants do not go on to use mindfulness skills in daily life. When participants share with the group the values-based actions they engaged in, they typically describe using skills of openness in response to the experiences that these actions bring up. Alongside these descriptions, participants may also share how they coped in ways consistent with their long-term strategies.

PRACTICE DEFUSION EXERCISES

In our experience, it can be tricky to present the concept of defusion to new workshop facilitators who don't have much experience with ACT. New facilitators often have several mistaken views about using defusion:

- That it is a way of convincing people that their thoughts are inaccurate

- That it is a way of being free from unhelpful or unwanted thoughts

- That it is a lasting change, and people need to work hard to achieve it

These ideas are probably influenced by the ways many people view the unusual experiences associated with psychosis: that these experiences should be controlled or gotten rid of in some way. Similarly, many people feel that the presence of negative and self-critical thoughts is a problem that needs to be solved. When training facilitators in the types of defusion we use in the workshops, exploring these ideas is a useful way to begin.

First, *defusion* is a way of observing thoughts, images, and memories that allows people to respond to mental experiences as *experiences* rather than *guides to action*. The passengers on the bus metaphor is a good way to orient facilitators to these types of responses, as it illustrates the challenge before us all: life's events shape us to have certain mental experiences, which we can respond to as though they are important guides to follow. We have a learned ability to derive relations between experiences, and our mind is a meaning-making machine. We attribute meaning to experience even when it may be self-defeating, may be mistaken, or may expand the ways that we suffer.

The passengers on the bus metaphor helps facilitators learn experientially that trying to change our experiences directly can be costly in terms of values-based action (that is, we fight with the bus's passengers). In ACT terms, we talk about life working by addition rather than subtraction: we do not unlearn what we already know and experience; instead, we can only elaborate on the meaning our mind creates. By noticing and becoming more aware of this process, we learn from our experience and respond in more flexible ways.

This is the key process that we want facilitators to notice when they run the workshop: Can they be aware of when participants are responding to internal experiences (passengers) in flexible ways? This may happen when the passengers on the bus exercise is acted out; when participants share with others their noticing experiences in the committed action activity; or when participants share "aha" moments, in which participants discover that they don't need to respond to experiences in the usual way. We want facilitators to acknowledge these moments of greater psychological flexibility and to resist the urge to overcomplicate the moments by adding more explanation.

GET IN CONTACT WITH VALUES AS DIRECTIONS AND COMMIT TO ACTION

We link commitment to action with chosen life directions (values) in the training sessions. For facilitators we typically need to unpack the concept of values. We do this by using the compass metaphor (Hayes et al., 1999; see chapter 2). The metaphor highlights the difference between goals and values and the idea of abstracted, broader purpose as guides for choices and actions. We demonstrate the key exercises used in the workshops and encourage facilitators to use their own life experiences, goals, and purposes when doing them. We discuss how *values* are like directions in life we want to move toward, whereas *goals* are things we want to achieve or complete. Within the compass metaphor, a value is like heading west, whereas goals are the locations along the way that indicate we are heading in that direction.

In the training sessions, we discuss the difference between getting married and being loving. If you want to be loving and caring, that's a value—it's ongoing. You want to behave that way for the rest of your life, and in any moment you have a choice: you can act on your value or neglect it. If you want to get married, that's a goal. It is something that you can achieve even if you neglect the values around being loving and caring.

We usually draw attention to the quality of vulnerability that frequently comes with connecting with valued directions. This is best demonstrated when facilitators use their own experiences of connecting with and sharing valued directions, choices, and actions. Trainers can help facilitators notice how valuing can evoke feelings and thoughts that invite struggle, and how the willingness and awareness skills (noticing, observing, making room for experiences as they are) can enable them to contact these experiences.

It can be useful to have facilitators link valued directions with actions they can take in the near future (whether it be later that day, during the week, or during the later training sessions). This link can then form useful material for reflecting on the process of committed action, which they will then promote in the workshops.

PROVIDE AN OPPORTUNITY TO PRACTICE EXERCISES AND GIVE GENERAL GUIDANCE

In the training sessions, facilitators can try out the exercises and learn the ways that work best for introducing noticing, willingness, and values construction. After an experienced facilitator (if there is one) has demonstrated the exercises, we encourage facilitators to pair up or form small groups to practice them. They should approach the group practice in a way that fosters learning—taking incremental steps toward running the workshops with fidelity—rather than create a pressured environment. Facilitators should encourage any behaviors that are consistent with the workshop program, and they should experiment with how they present the material, seek feedback, and foster noticing and curiosity. What follows are general bits of guidance to offer during the training sessions.

Keep the ACT for recovery workshops focused. The workshops should be skills focused. We encourage participants to consider the ideas and skills that are being presented, and to try them out in their own lives. We encourage participants to *trust their own experience* about the usefulness of the workshops. This means that, compared to other groups that may be primarily about sharing life stories and providing support, the ACT for recovery workshops are more focused on exercises and reflections about these elements. It is the job of the facilitators to keep this focus in mind and, when necessary, to redirect the group back to the skills and exercises. At times this will mean respectfully interrupting participants and finding ways to link the discussion back to the broader group goals.

Create a group environment that promotes sharing and exploration while not debating about, arguing about, or convincing participants of the merits of ACT. The ACT for recovery workshops are about an experiential form of learning. This can be contrasted with groups that have an educational purpose or are about helping participants correct or fix their perspectives. The ACT model is a pragmatic approach, not something to have debates about, or to try to convince workshop participants to take on board as "the answer."

This means that we encourage facilitators to present the exercises and ideas as potentially useful, as things for the participants to try out and see. As much as possible, we lead the sessions in a way that minimizes arguments and contradictions. The aim is to find examples within the participants' and facilitators' lives that illustrate the usefulness of an open, aware, and active approach to living.

This approach also means that facilitators avoid a problem-solving stance, wherein participant actions could be cast as problematic or in error. Instead, as much as possible, facilitators should seek to understand why participants make the choices that they do, to validate the purposes of this, and to promote linking actions to valued directions. This focus necessitates using noticing and willingness as starting points.

It is a goal-driven world, and we are trying to link people to valuing. Some participants interpret the values-construction work in ACT for recovery as being consistent with the type of goal setting that sometimes occurs in mental health settings: where the care coordinator or case manager sets goals for the client to achieve. This unilateral form of goal setting, where participants frequently cannot link with their valued directions, is inconsistent with the approach taken in the workshop sessions.

The values-construction approach taken in ACT for recovery can hopefully be contrasted with other forms of goal setting. While we are all drivers on our bus of life, sometimes we are unclear about where we are going, or we have passengers tell us where it is important to go, for long periods. Stepping back from these goals by practicing noticing, willingness, and distancing can sometimes help us create the conditions to get in touch with what matters, or (when things are unclear) it can help us spend time choosing life directions to try out. Values are larger than goals.

What to do when participants have not completed committed action activities. It is common for participants, especially those recovering from serious mental illness, to have trouble with or not complete committed action activities. These are opportunities for the facilitators to start shaping a psychologically flexible stance by engaging participants in observing and noticing skills. In the small group work, where committed actions are identified and plans are made, facilitators can encourage participants to bring their noticing skills to the process. Even when participants have not completed a committed action activity, facilitators can use this opportunity to help them notice what happened, which passengers got in the way (barriers), and what it is like to share the experience in the workshop. In ACT for recovery we are more interested in the *process of valuing* than the outcomes: by engaging participants in noticing this process, it may increase the odds that they use these skills the next time an opportunity arises to act on values.

In this way no one fails when it comes to doing committed action activities. Whether one accomplishes them or not becomes material to notice; it becomes a way to connect with the shared (challenging) experience of being human and trying to do things that matter.

It's also important to remember that the workshops are designed to progressively shape behavior over time. So, when participants initially struggle to identify values or actions linked to values, or they find it hard to complete committed action tasks, a skilled facilitator will focus on broader learning as it occurs over the course of the group, rather than attempting to push learning within a session when participants may not be quite ready.

Summary

In this chapter, we described a range of ways to improve your skills as an ACT for recovery workshop facilitator, as well as ideas for how to support other facilitators in this goal. A key goal for workshop facilitators is to become increasingly fluent with the ACT model, understanding it as a set of practices for and ways of responding in the moment, so that workshop sessions promote flexible, experiential learning. Working in this recovery-oriented way involves plenty of practice and feedback. For these reasons, it is ideal to develop these skills as a team. We hope that the tips and advice in this chapter, based on our experiences of training facilitators, will help you facilitate engaging and effective workshops.

CHAPTER 6

Running Successful and Effective Workshops

Supervision and Evaluation

Providing training to facilitators is only one part of ensuring that the ACT for recovery workshops provide high quality experiences for participants. We think it is good practice to provide facilitators with ongoing supervision as well. This will strengthen their skills for running the workshops and deepen their familiarity with the model. Supervision is a good way to troubleshoot issues that arise in the workshops, including group dynamics that may maintain rigidity and inflexibility. In supervision, you can discuss what's been happening in the workshops, engage in problem solving, role-play challenging exchanges, and help the facilitators further develop their skills.

This chapter is also concerned with evaluating the workshops. Being able to demonstrate whether participants benefited is an important consideration for both participants and services. In many settings treatment providers are required to demonstrate that their interventions improve clients' lives and are acceptable and safe. We will discuss ways to evaluate ACT for recovery workshops that will enable you to judge whether the program benefited participants. Evaluation can be done using available outcome measures to track well-being, valued actions, recovery stages, quality of life (validated to be used with people with psychosis), and personal improvements with individualized goals. We will describe the approach we took for our ACT for Recovery study, as well as the clinical measures being used in routine clinical practice.

Supervision

Engaging facilitators in supervision (consultation) ensures that the workshops are high quality learning experiences and that the facilitators are supported in their role. Supervision is most important when facilitators are first learning how to lead the workshops; it helps them develop ACT skills and maintains adherence to the group protocol.

Supervision of Workshop Facilitators

We suggest that you arrange regular supervision meetings with the team of facilitators who is leading the workshops. If you have peer-support facilitators in your program, it is useful to involve them in these meetings, too; however, you may want a separate supervision process for them (see below) or for the professional facilitators to offer this support.

We recommend that supervisors include the following practices in group supervision meetings:

- Spell out what facilitators should expect from the meetings so they feel supported in their development of competencies. This includes discussing how you will offer constructive criticism.

- Review how the group sessions have been, including positive and negative experiences with leading the workshops.

- Have facilitators share their knowledge and understanding of the workshop protocol.

- Practice the exercises to fine-tune delivery.

- Role-play experiential methods to problem solve group challenges.

- Seek feedback from the facilitators about their experience of the meeting.

In our experience, meeting for at least an hour is optimal, and meeting after every two workshop sessions is the minimum, depending on facilitator need. An hour offers enough time to raise questions, give feedback, problem solve, and practice exercises.

Consistent with the agreed-upon best practices of supervision and what we know about learning interventions, we recommend that, as much as possible, you make the supervision meetings a mixture of support, problem solving, and experiential learning (rather than simply having them be about reporting on how the workshop sessions went or discussing practical issues). To support experiential learning, it is optimal for facilitators to describe what happened in the workshop sessions and how they responded to the group process, to encourage them to share areas of concern, and to use role-playing and other experiential methods to further develop the facilitators' skills (Morris & Bilich-Eric, 2017).

How to Offer Supervision to Peer-Support Facilitators

In the ACT for Recovery study we engaged peer-support facilitators to cofacilitate the workshops. Their inclusion offered many advantages (see chapter 4). The model of workshop delivery that we endorse is one that offers clear expectations of these facilitators. As we described in chapter 4, to meet these expectations, and for the workshop experience to be a positive one for both them and the participants, it is essential that peer-support facilitators are well supported. Supervision meetings are a good way to offer support.

We think the supervision meetings should be similar to those of the facilitators who are health professionals. By this we mean there should be formal supervision meetings (as described above) that run at least an hour. In the meetings the workshop leader and facilitators should have the opportunity to review the workshop process, to practice skills, and to prepare for future sessions.

It is important to consider expectations and structure in offering supervision to peer-support facilitators. Foremost, peer-support facilitators may not have supervision experience, so setting expectations for the purpose and format of the meetings is very useful. Also, providing facilitators with a rationale for supervision, that it is about providing them support so they can do the best job they can for the workshop participants, is usually a good way to reassure them and gain their interest and cooperation.

In supervision sessions, supervisors need to be mindful of their expectations of the peer-support facilitator role and should consider the following:

- Lack of professional knowledge or training

- The tension that can develop between being a workshop facilitator and being a person who has experienced mental health treatment

- Feelings that arise from facilitating workshops or participating in supervision, particularly experiences of feeling confused, overwhelmed, or criticized

CONSIDERING POTENTIAL LACK OF PROFESSIONAL KNOWLEDGE OR TRAINING

Peer-support facilitators bring expertise about the experience of recovering from mental health problems, and their perspective can support workshop participants as they try out the psychological flexibility skills promoted in the workshops. The peer-support facilitator's presence and communication about recovery can be a powerful influence on the success of the group process.

However, a peer's perspective has limited scope in some areas. For example, peer supporters are unlikely to have broad knowledge of evidence-based understandings of mental health and well-being; of how health and social care systems operate; or of the options—beyond those of the workshop—available to respond to the needs of the workshop participants (such as being able to refer participants, in an informed way, to services and supports that they need).

It is also important for clinicians running the workshops to maintain clarity about the responsibilities peer-support facilitators have with respect to the participants. Sometimes workshop participants lean on peer-support facilitators to respond to issues that are the clinician's responsibility. For example, when a participant arrives to a session in crisis, or if his or her mental state or level of risk has recently worsened, the peer supporter should not take on responsibility for managing these issues, as this is a clinician's responsibility.

It is also essential in health care settings to consider what governs the conduct of peer-support facilitators. In the ACT for Recovery study we recruited the facilitators, paying them for the time they spent training, cofacilitating workshops, and participating in supervision. Because we recruited them from a service-user involvement register, a voluntary listing of peer workers that is managed by our health service, they had already been interviewed and vetted and had agreed to standards of conduct as part of the contract to be on the register. It also meant that they had already received some orientation into working in a health service setting. It is useful to consider how these recruitment processes and governance procedures operate in your setting, so you can establish clear roles and responsibilities for facilitators, both health professionals and peers.

"HOW AM I AN EXPERT?"

Because they are experts by experience, peer-support facilitators sometimes find themselves in the position of managing the tension between providing this expertise and engaging in their own mental health care. Sometimes they may feel fraudulent, as if they haven't been all that successful in their personal recovery. This may lead them to question their own contributions to the workshop process.

We think these concerns should be directly discussed in supervision. The ACT model offers a shared perspective that the supervisor and facilitators can take: the normality and universality of suffering, how the skills practiced in the workshops are applicable across a range of situations, and that the intention of offering peer support is to encourage participants and facilitators to use these skills (not just in periods of greater distress, or when one is recovering from an episode or a mental health problem, but as a regular feature of living life well). The perspective the supervisor can put forth is that the peer-support facilitators are sharing their recovery experiences, and, by being visible to the workshop participants, they are offering something valuable in its own right. The supervisor can offer encouragement by pointing out times when the peer-support facilitator led exercises and shared experiences in ways that were useful in the workshop sessions, leading to productive discussion and feedback or perhaps enhanced disclosure and openness from workshop participants.

PROVIDING A SAFE SPACE FOR SUPERVISION

Facilitating workshops can be challenging. There will be times when, despite the best planning and intentions, a workshop session will not go as expected, or it will involve discussions that leave the peer-support facilitator confused or overwhelmed. Sometimes participants criticize facilitators, or they don't accept the limits established by the workshop rules.

Supervision serves an important function on these occasions. By providing a supportive space to discuss this material, and for the supervisor to validate a facilitator's experiences, the opportunity to strengthen flexible responding arises. This can be done through discussion, by reviewing audio recordings, or by role-playing the interactions. Establishing in supervision the expectation that group work involves these feelings and responses, and that there is value in openly discussing them, can go a long way to building the capacity of facilitators to handle the complexity of the sessions.

Helping Facilitators Run ACT for Recovery Workshops with Fidelity

For any intervention based on empirical evaluation, it is important to consider how to support the facilitators so they can deliver it with fidelity. In this section, we will describe ways to track fidelity and provide feedback to facilitators, and we'll give you tips about this process in practice.

Fidelity involves both *adherence* to the intervention (doing the key tasks involved, along with making sure that you are not doing things that are incompatible with the intervention) and *competence* (doing the intervention in a way that is impactful, with well-timed and sensitive use of techniques). Fidelity is a key element when doing research studies of interventions, and we think it is also important when delivering groups in regular settings. Facilitators may be doing the key tasks of the ACT model, but they may not show competence, as their responses to participants may not be ACT consistent. The workshops are more than "just" running people through exercises and giving them committed action activities to do.

The ACT for recovery workshop is intended to be a short-term, manualized intervention. This means that it should require less facilitator skill than, say, engaging a participant in individually tailored acceptance and commitment therapy. In our research studies, we typically led the workshop with a team of facilitators, including an experienced person and a couple of people who had recently been trained to facilitate the workshop (for example, a peer-support facilitator). This meant that in each workshop there was a skilled facilitator with the capacity, based on depth of knowledge and skill with ACT, to respond to unusual or challenging interactions. We appreciate that not every setting will have this level of expertise on hand. We think that because most of our facilitators were not highly trained or professionally educated ACT therapists, that it is possible to run the workshops without a lot of expertise, which may make delivering the workshops feasible in many settings.

The ACTs of ACT

We have tracked fidelity using what we call the ACTs of ACT Fidelity Measure (see figure 2). It reflects the relationship between adherence and competence.

Figure 2. The ACTs of ACT Fidelity Measure

Workshop session number: _____ **Date:** _____

For the workshop session, please rate for the presence of each of the components below.

For each component that is *present*, please rate how appropriate it is for this stage of therapy, and then rate group responsiveness to this component.

ACT therapeutic stance	How present in this session?	How appropriate for this session?	Group responsiveness?
	0 = Not at all 1 = Minimal 2 = Satisfactory 3 = High 4 = Very high	0 = Inappropriate 1 = Minimally 2 = Satisfactory 3 = Highly 4 = Very high	0 = Unresponsive 1 = Minimal 2 = Satisfactory 3 = High 4 = Very high
Developing acceptance and willingness/undermining experiential control	How present in this session?	How appropriate for this session?	Group responsiveness?
	0 = Not at all 1 = Minimal 2 = Satisfactory 3 = High 4 = Very high	0 = Inappropriate 1 = Minimally 2 = Satisfactory 3 = Highly 4 = Very high	0 = Unresponsive 1 = Minimal 2 = Satisfactory 3 = High 4 = Very high
Undermining cognitive fusion	How present in this session?	How appropriate for this session?	Group responsiveness?
	0 = Not at all 1 = Minimal 2 = Satisfactory 3 = High 4 = Very high	0 = Inappropriate 1 = Minimally 2 = Satisfactory 3 = Highly 4 = Very high	0 = Unresponsive 1 = Minimal 2 = Satisfactory 3 = High 4 = Very high
Getting in contact with the present moment	How present in this session?	How appropriate for this session?	Group responsiveness?
	0 = Not at all 1 = Minimal 2 = Satisfactory 3 = High 4 = Very high	0 = Inappropriate 1 = Minimally 2 = Satisfactory 3 = Highly 4 = Very high	0 = Unresponsive 1 = Minimal 2 = Satisfactory 3 = High 4 = Very high
Distinguishing the conceptualized self from self-as-context	How present in this session?	How appropriate for this session?	Group responsiveness?
	0 = Not at all 1 = Minimal 2 = Satisfactory 3 = High 4 = Very high	0 = Inappropriate 1 = Minimally 2 = Satisfactory 3 = Highly 4 = Very high	0 = Unresponsive 1 = Minimal 2 = Satisfactory 3 = High 4 = Very high

Defining valued directions	How present in this session?	How appropriate for this session?	Group responsiveness?
	0 = Not at all 1 = Minimal 2 = Satisfactory 3 = High 4 = Very high	0 = Inappropriate 1 = Minimally 2 = Satisfactory 3 = Highly 4 = Very high	0 = Unresponsive 1 = Minimal 2 = Satisfactory 3 = High 4 = Very high
Building patterns of committed action	How present in this session?	How appropriate for this session?	Group responsiveness?
	0 = Not at all 1 = Minimal 2 = Satisfactory 3 = High 4 = Very high	0 = Inappropriate 1 = Minimally 2 = Satisfactory 3 = Highly 4 = Very high	0 = Unresponsive 1 = Minimal 2 = Satisfactory 3 = High 4 = Very high

ACT-Inconsistent Techniques/Proscribed Behaviors	How Present in This Session?
Did the facilitator explain the "meaning" of paradoxes or metaphors (possibly to develop "insight")?	0 = Not at all 1 = Minimal 2 = Moderate 3 = High 4 = Very high
Did the facilitator engage in criticism, judgment, or taking a "one-up" position?	0 = Not at all 1 = Minimal 2 = Moderate 3 = High 4 = Very high
Did the facilitator argue with, lecture, coerce, or attempt to convince the participant?	0 = Not at all 1 = Minimal 2 = Moderate 3 = High 4 = Very high
Did the facilitator substitute his or her opinions for the participant's genuine experience of what is working or not working?	0 = Not at all 1 = Minimal 2 = Moderate 3 = High 4 = Very high

Did the facilitator model the need to resolve contradictory or difficult ideas, feelings, memories, and the like?	0 = Not at all 1 = Minimal 2 = Moderate 3 = High 4 = Very high
Evidence for delusional beliefs: Did the facilitator assess the evidence the participant uses to support his or her delusional beliefs?	0 = Not at all 1 = Minimal 2 = Moderate 3 = High 4 = Very high
Validity testing/behavioral experiments: Did the facilitator encourage the participant to (1) engage in specific behaviors for the purpose of testing the validity of his or her beliefs, or (2) make explicit predictions about external events so that the outcomes of those events could serve as tests of those predictions, or (3) review the outcome of previous validity tests?	0 = Not at all 1 = Minimal 2 = Moderate 3 = High 4 = Very high
Verbal challenge of delusions: Did the facilitator challenge the participant's beliefs through discussion?	0 = Not at all 1 = Minimal 2 = Moderate 3 = High 4 = Very high

Overall Rating

How would you rate the facilitator's performance *overall* in leading group ACT in this session?

0	1	2	3	4	5	6
Poor	Barely adequate	Mediocre	Satisfactory	Good	Very good	Excellent

ACT-CONSISTENT FACILITATOR BEHAVIORS

The first section of the ACTs of ACT Fidelity Measure describes the ACT-consistent behaviors we want the workshop facilitators to engage in. The group protocol (see part 2) describes both the content of the sessions, as well as the style the facilitators should use for the interactions. Indicating whether an ACT-consistent behavior is present in the session assesses adherence to the protocol, while rating the appropriateness of the ACT component assesses competence. Attending to the participants' responses to these behaviors is also part of assessing competence, in that doing so considers whether the facilitator carried out the component in a timely and skillful way.

ACT-INCONSISTENT FACILITATOR BEHAVIORS

The second part of the ACTs of ACT Fidelity Measure is a listing of proscribed facilitator behaviors. These behaviors are likely to work at cross-purposes with promoting the psychological flexibility of participants: they may (1) strengthen the idea that the content of participants' experiences needs to change, or is incorrect or wrong in some way; or they may (2) reinforce the view that participants need to respond to experiences by "testing them out," "working them out," or "understanding them." Instead, we want to encourage participants to respond to experiences by just observing or noticing them, nonjudgmentally. Holding lightly the idea of making sense of experiences is likely to lead to greater flexibility in how participants respond to them.

Typically, nonadherent responses occur when facilitators present ACT components at inopportune times, or when the interaction is about something other than promoting psychological flexibility skills. A couple of examples may help clarify.

- **Mistiming:** When facilitators present the possibilities of responding with willingness or defusing from thoughts outside of the broader purpose of making values-based choices and taking action, participants are likely to experience both options as invalidating or promoting inappropriate messages, such as "just ignore your thoughts" or "what your mind says does not matter." In our experience, starting with present-moment awareness and noticing, and exploring valuing as a way to connect with sources of motivation and meaning, are better ways to create a foundation from which participants can explore whether acceptance and defusion can help them live more consistently with their values.

- **Responding to content, rather than context:** There are times during the workshops when facilitators can get caught up by the content that participants describe. This can lead to responses that are about problem solving or "fixing," rather than about promoting flexibility. Responding to content in this way can also happen when facilitators become rigid in how they present the ACT model to participants, such as by presenting it as "the answer" or "the right way of doing things," rather than as a set of skills to experiment with. Facilitators can track this in the sessions by reflecting on whether they are taking an expert position in relation to participants instead of presenting and responding as equals. The process of groups can tolerate a fair degree of skepticism and questioning from participants: we want people to engage with the metaphors and ideas of the ACT model on their own terms. Sometimes it is going to be important for facilitators to "agree to disagree" with participants. This may especially be the case when participants express overvalued or delusional ideas during the workshop sessions. Facilitators need to check to make sure they are leading the groups with flexibility, too!

OPPORTUNITIES TO ASSESS FIDELITY

There are several ways to assess fidelity, including directly observing or recording (both audio and video) workshop sessions. Directly observing the sessions, possibly as a cofacilitator, is a good way to see if the facilitator engages in ACT-consistent and ACT-inconsistent behaviors, as well how workshop participants respond to these behaviors.

If workshop participants consent, audio recordings can be a useful way to assess fidelity. Facilitators can share session excerpts in supervision meetings to gain feedback on their performance and to review participant responses. Alternatively, the supervisor can listen to the audio recording before offering feedback, problem solving, and possibly role-playing alternative responses in supervision meetings.

Video recordings may be more difficult to organize, as workshop participants may be less willing to consent. However, video recordings provide an excellent way to assess both how facilitators present the workshop, as well as how participants respond to the material, including nonverbal responding (such as observations of how engaged the participants are, whether facilitators missed opportunities to respond, and so forth).

Regular supervision meetings (as discussed above), in which you give feedback to facilitators, are an essential part of the supervision process and of promoting fidelity. We think constructive feedback and modeling (the supervisor demonstrating various ways to run exercises and handle interactions) are the best ways to ensure fidelity.

Evaluating Workshops

In this section we describe ways to evaluate the ACT for recovery workshop program in your setting. We outline why we think assessing the program is useful and the types of measures and feedback to use, including assessments that can be tailored to the personal recovery of each participant.

Why Evaluate the Workshop Program in Your Setting?

In general, we have found that it is a good idea to ask participants about how they felt about any intervention we offer. We recommend that, in planning to run the ACT for recovery workshops, you establish a method to evaluate how useful the sessions were for the participants.

We hope that by evaluating the workshop program you will discover what works best for participants. Seeking their feedback will assist you as you adjust and change ACT for recovery so it can be useful in your setting. Evaluating the workshop program will help you determine whether the workshops are achieving their intended purpose: to improve participants' well-being by increasing their engagement in values-based actions.

Along with the workshop participants, in many settings there are a variety of stakeholders, including referring professionals and agencies, the management of your service, and the families and caregivers of workshop participants, who are interested in whether the workshops you offer actually help people. Being able to provide them summaries of the evaluations you've done will help them understand what the program is about and what to expect for the workshop participants.

Considerations for Using Assessment Measures

It is useful to be pragmatic when doing assessments in routine practice. While a range of measures can be used in research studies in order to test a variety of predictions, measuring predictions is not the purpose in service evaluations. In routine service delivery, the focus of assessment should be upon demonstrating whether the program is beneficial to the participants. We suggest choosing measures that are validated for the population you work with, are sensitive to change, and are open source and publicly available. (For a broader discussion of the development of measures to evaluate ACT for people with psychosis, we recommend Farhall, Shawyer, Thomas, & Morris, 2013.)

We also recommend that you consider how much assessment workshop participants may tolerate. You don't want workshop preassessment to be so burdensome that it puts participants off from coming to the workshops! Lengthy assessment measures or interviews are too much for some people recovering from psychosis to tolerate, so it is better to use briefer measures. This has certainly been a consideration in acute settings (see chapter 3 for a discussion). Using measures that have been validated for the population with which you are working (either for people with psychosis, or for caregivers) is important; the validation ensures that any changes you find are reliable, valid, and applicable to your participant group.

Finally, for self-report questionnaires we recommend using open-source measures that are publicly available. The advantage of these measures is that they are free and cost little to produce in paper form. Also, because they are publicly available, if you wish you are free to develop electronic versions (an app on a tablet or an online survey).

Types of Measures and Feedback to Use

ACT is an approach that aims to promote well-being, purpose, and quality of life using psychological flexibility skills, so these are the types of outcomes and processes to evaluate following the workshops. We therefore suggest that you seek two broad sets of measures (outcomes and processes) and feedback from the workshop participants.

Outcome Measures

It's important to assess outcome measures, including well-being, interference from symptoms and problems, quality of life, level of activity, and engagement in personal recovery.

WELL-BEING

A key outcome from the workshops is that they improve participant well-being. Several measures for this have been validated for people with psychosis.

The Clinical Outcomes in Routine Evaluation–Outcome Measure (CORE–OM): This public-domain thirty-four-point self-measure of psychological distress is made up of four domains: well-being (four items), symptoms (twelve items), functioning (twelve items), and risk (six items). It has been used in a variety of psychological therapy evaluations for people with psychosis (for example, Chadwick et al., 2016; Jolley, Garety, et al., 2015; Waller et al., 2013). You can download the CORE–OM for free (http://www.coreims.co.uk).

The Clinical Outcomes in Routine Evaluation–10 (CORE–10; Barkham et al., 2013): This short form of the CORE–OM, using ten items drawn from the measure, is used when the CORE–OM is regarded as too lengthy. The items cover anxiety (two), depression (two), trauma (one), physical problems (one), functioning (three—day to day, close relationships, social relationships), and risk to self (one). The CORE–10 has also been used to evaluate psychological approaches with people with psychosis (for example, Owen, Sellwood, Kan, Murray, & Sarsam, 2015; Jolley, Garety, et al., 2015).

The Warwick-Edinburgh Mental Well-Being Scale (WEMWBS; Tennant et al., 2007): This fourteen-item scale covers both the feeling and functioning aspects of mental well-being. It has been found to be a valid measure of mental well-being across a diverse range of clinical problems (Stewart-Brown et al., 2011), including with people with psychosis and those sensitive to change (Jolley, Onwumere, et al., 2015). You can download it for free at http://www2.warwick.ac.uk/fac/med/research/platform/wemwbs.

INTERFERENCE FROM SYMPTOMS AND PROBLEMS

ACT interventions reduce the interference from symptoms and problems that participants perceive. One measures assesses this.

The Sheehan Disability Scale (SDS; D. V. Sheehan, Harnett-Sheehan, & Raj, 1996): This three-item measure, adapted from the Sheehan Disability Scales (D. V. Sheehan, 1983), looks at functional impairment in three domains: work/study, social life/leisure activities, and family life/home responsibilities. The client rates how much their difficulties have interfered with these areas of life in the past week using a ten-point visual analogue scale. The SDS has good psychometric properties and is sensitive to treatment effects (K. H. Sheehan & Sheehan, 2008).

QUALITY OF LIFE

ACT interventions improve quality of life for participants, which the following measure assesses.

Manchester Short Assessment of Quality of Life (MANSA; Priebe, Huxley, Knight, & Evans, 1999): This sixteen-item scale assesses satisfaction with life domains (for example, employment/training, finances, friendships, accommodations, family relationships, physical and mental health). Participants rate items on a seven-point scale; the item average is the MANSA summary score (higher scores suggest greater quality of life). A range of studies of people with psychosis have used the MANSA as a quality-of-life scale (for example, McCrone, Craig, Power, & Garety, 2010; Theodore et al., 2012).

ACTIVITY LEVELS

The ACT workshops have a focus on increasing values-based action, and for many participants this is about increasing activity in general, including the range and complexity of the activities.

The Time Budget Measure (Jolley et al., 2006): This measure takes the form of a weeklong diary, wherein each day is divided into four time blocks. The participants are asked to describe what they have been doing in each of these time blocks, which the interviewer then rates on a five-point scale (ranging from low activity, such as sitting, sleeping, and so forth, to demanding activities requiring planning and motivation, such as work, studying, and so on). The overall score provides a measure of activity for the week.

ENGAGEMENT IN PERSONAL RECOVERY

The ACT workshops are designed to increase participants' engagement in their own personal recovery.

Questionnaire About the Process of Recovery (QPR; Neil et al., 2009): This twenty-two-item measure asks people about recovery in ways that are meaningful to them. There are two subscales: intrapersonal tasks involved in recovery and interpersonal factors that assist recovery. Higher scores are indicative of recovery. Recent evaluations of the QPR suggest that it has reasonable psychometric properties, and a fifteen-item short-form version is available (J. Williams et al., 2015).

Process Measures

It is also useful to assess the processes of change associated with ACT, such as mindfulness, nonjudgment of experiences, values-based action, and psychological flexibility.

The Southampton Mindfulness Questionnaire (SMQ; Chadwick et al., 2008): This sixteen-item scale assesses an individual's relationship with distressing thoughts and images and the degree to which he or she responds mindfully to distressing experiences. The measure includes items about accepting difficult thoughts and images and letting difficult thoughts pass without reacting. The SMQ has good psychometric qualities (Chadwick et al., 2008).

The Cognitive Fusion Questionnaire (CFQ; Gillanders et al., 2014): This seven-item scale is designed to measure the degree to which a person nonjudgmentally engages experiences, assessing the extent to which internal experiences govern and influence behavior.

The Valuing Questionnaire (VQ; Smout et al., 2014): This eight-item values (general rather than domain specific) measure captures two facets of valued living: progress in engaging in valued directions and obstructions to this.

The Acceptance and Action Questionnaire–2 (AAQ–2; Bond et al., 2011): This seven-item questionnaire is designed to measure psychological flexibility. High scores suggest greater acceptance of mental experiences and persistence with life goals in the face of these experiences. The AAQ–2 has excellent psychometric properties.

Feedback About the Workshop Experience

It is very useful to seek participants' opinions about their group experience, both during sessions and, in a formal way, after the final workshop session.

PARTICIPANT SATISFACTION

Using general consumer-satisfaction methods, you can gain feedback about whether participants found the workshop acceptable and helpful and whether they would recommend it to others.

We recommend that you use a series of questions based on a measure like the Client Satisfaction Questionnaire–8 (CSQ–8; Larsen, Attkisson, Hargreaves, & Nguyen, 1979), modified to be relevant to the workshop. (Appendix A15 is an example of what we used in our studies.) Participants score the items of this measure on a four-point Likert scale, with a higher score indicating greater satisfaction. In addition, it is useful to ask participants open-ended questions about what they found most helpful in the workshops, what they found least helpful, and what they would recommend be changed in future workshops. Finally, we suggest using the Family and Friends Test (NHS England, 2013); you can do this by simply asking participants to rate their answer to the following question on a scale of 1 (extremely likely) to 5 (extremely unlikely): How likely are you to recommend the workshops to friends and family if they need similar help?

Constructive feedback is very helpful. In our experience, a lot can be learned from inviting participants to share their criticisms of the workshops, areas that they felt weren't so useful, and any moments or experiences that were off-putting. In a number of important ways, the group protocol presented later in this book is the result of what we learned from participants about what worked for them and what didn't.

Summary

Chapters 5 and 6 focused on how you can train facilitators to run the ACT for recovery workshops, provide supervision to ensure their fidelity to the intervention is supported, and evaluate the impact of the workshops.

We believe that ACT for recovery workshops should involve these components. The time you spend setting up these supporting features is worthwhile, as they will ensure that both participants and facilitators have the best group experience possible.

PART 2

Treatment Manual

Introduction to ACT for Psychosis Recovery Workshop Protocol

Written with Natasha Avery

This part of the manual provides a complete protocol for running the ACT for recovery workshops in community group settings. The protocol comprises a ninety-minute taster session and four two-hour sessions. We also include two, two-hour booster sessions.

The workshops are designed to be run as closed groups with six to twelve participants and two to three facilitators. We recommend that participants are at a similar stage of recovery (for example, first-episode psychosis clients or clients with longer-term, more complex needs). We suggest this because we have noticed that participants in the early stages of their psychosis tend to be more withdrawn and nervous about attending groups. We have also noticed that they are sometimes more invested in approaches to control and eliminate symptoms. With this group of participants, we believe it is important to attend to their needs, including being engaged, flexible, and hands-on, such as managing shyness. Participants with more established psychosis are often more accustomed to attending groups, and thus they are more likely to present as being confident. However, at times we have noticed that people who have lived with psychosis longer are often more stuck. For these reasons we feel that groups that are homogenous in terms of recovery are more helpful and can provide a sense of universality, which is also valued within the workshops.

We used this protocol as part of a research study in community mental health settings, one group with people experiencing psychosis (see chapter 1) and one with caregivers of people with psychosis (see chapter 2), and the results were promising. We used the same protocol for both groups of participants, apart from adding the reservoir metaphor to the caregiver workshops and the different videos (shown in the sessions) of George and Paul, which are clearly marked within the protocol. You can download these videos at http://www.

actforpsychosis.com. If you prefer to make your own videos, the transcripts of both are included as appendix A6 and appendix A7.

We provide guidelines for the amount of time to spend on each exercise. However, depending on the needs of workshop members, you may wish to adjust the amount devoted to different elements of each session. Depending on the group, you may need to devote more time to particular exercises. If a session runs too long and you can't fit everything in, you can move the remaining elements to the next session. You may choose to increase the number of sessions beyond four, if required. We also provide suggestions for how to facilitate certain exercises, as well as tips from our own observations of running many ACT for recovery workshops.

The presentation of the sessions follows the same general format. At the start of each we provide a general outline of the session's main elements, including estimated time frames. We provide a list of materials needed for each session as well. For each exercise we highlight its aim and suggest how its presentation can unfold. Throughout these sessions we provide samples of dialogue that you may find useful to use in your own sessions.

Preworkshop Orientation

We recommend meeting with each potential participant prior to the start of the workshop in order to provide an overview of the workshop sessions, discuss goals for attending, and address any concerns about the workshop. We have found that this process builds engagement from an early stage. We have also found it useful to problem solve with participants any issues they anticipate, including worries about speaking in a group, punctuality, or learning and reading needs.

We designed the taster session to be an informal introduction to some of the elements of the ACT for recovery workshops. From it participants can then decide whether to attend the main workshop program.

In-Session Suggestions

We recommend minimizing the us-versus-them atmosphere by seating workshop facilitators among the participants. We also encourage all facilitators to participate in the group exercises when they are not taking the lead.

Self-disclosure can be helpful, when appropriate, and we encourage facilitators to self-disclose in sessions. For example, if a facilitator was feeling particularly tired one day, she could mention that this was a passenger she had been struggling with; or, a facilitator may disclose that he had been struggling with anxiety passengers prior to an important presentation. This sort of self-disclosure should feel appropriate for the context of the workshop (see chapter 5 for more discussion). We recommend providing light refreshments and having a short (ten to fifteen minutes) break halfway through the session.

Each session in the protocol provides details about required materials and worksheets. See appendix A for prompt sheets for specific exercises that you can photocopy and use in the workshops, and appendix B for the worksheets used in each session. We recommend providing each participant with a folder or binder in which to keep the workshop materials. Participants can decide whether they want to take their folder or binder home each week or leave it with group facilitators.

We provide all participants with recordings of the mindfulness exercises, either on a compact disc, USB stick, or via a link for download. You can access the recordings at http://www.actforpsychosis.com. We recommend that you record your own mindfulness exercises, which can follow the guided mindfulness instructions in appendix A.

Between-Session Phone Calls

We ask participants if it would be okay for us to call them in between the sessions. We explain that we wouldn't use this as an excuse to "check up" on them to see if they had engaged in their committed action. Instead we frame these brief phone calls as a way of "checking in" with them, asking how they found the workshop that week or if they noticed any passengers over the week, and of supporting them in their efforts to respond differently to the passengers. Feedback has indicated that participants value the phone calls and that they serve as helpful reminders about committed action and encourage attendance of the next session.

Booster Sessions

The booster sessions are designed to act as refreshers for the skills taught in the workshop. We suggest running them over two consecutive weeks eight weeks after the workshop ends. Most participants have attended at least one or both of the booster sessions and reported finding the refreshers helpful.

Final Message

We hope you enjoy facilitating the ACT for recovery workshops as much as we have!

Taster Session

The introduction, or taster session, is intended to introduce the participants—whether clients or caregivers—to the series of workshops. In addition to helping the members of the group feel oriented to the space and the format, the facilitator will introduce the concept of values (using the passengers on the bus metaphor) and barriers to values. Facilitators will introduce the idea of automatic pilot and lead the group through the "mindfulness of breath and body" exercise. The session closes with a discussion of dates for future workshops. The following session outline suggests an order for the topics and time frames. As always, the times given for each segment are approximate.

Timeline

Welcome and introduction	10 minutes
Introducing values (active)	20 minutes
Introducing the passengers on the bus metaphor	25 minutes
Mindfulness exercise (aware)	25 minutes
Closing the session	10 minutes

Materials You'll Need

- Whiteboard
- Paper and pens
- Marker pens
- Flip chart
- Refreshments

Welcome and Introduction

Aim: To make participants feel welcome and to highlight the purpose of the workshop sessions by working through the key points on the whiteboard.

Welcome participants to the taster session of the ACT for recovery workshops. Explain that the session will run for approximately one and a half hours with a short break halfway through. Introduce housekeeping issues (for example, fire escapes, bathrooms, and so forth). Facilitators should introduce themselves and their roles and write their names on a name badge. Ask participants also to wear name badges.

Explain that the taster session aims to give people a chance to find out what the workshops are about and to try out some of the exercises. Emphasize that these are "skills workshops" rather than therapeutic groups, so you will be encouraging them to talk about how they find the practices and what they notice from the exercises, rather than discussing personal issues in depth. Explain that there won't be enough time for this.

> For workshops for caregivers, it's important to highlight that caring for someone with mental health problems can be extremely rewarding, but it also can be stressful and burdensome and can have a significant impact on relationships; and explain how the workshops can help people discover what matters to them and how to use that knowledge to set goals and to take actions that enrich their lives.

During the taster sessions for both caregivers and clients, introduce what these groups are about:

- Developing life direction
- Increasing awareness of obstacles
- Learning the skills of open, aware, and active in order to respond more effectively to obstacles
- Connecting with each other and having fun

Dialogue Example

Here are some of the key points for this series of workshops. We'll be exploring each of these areas session by session.

Introduce the Reservoir Metaphor (Caregiver Workshops)

At this point in sessions for caregivers, it's time to introduce the reservoir metaphor as a way of identifying how important it is for them to maintain their own well-being, and how the workshops may be useful for this. If this is a session for clients, skip this metaphor.

The Reservoir Metaphor

We all have "emotional reservoirs" of different types. Some supply energy, others supply health or well-being. When the reservoirs are full, we can maintain our energy or well-being, even in times of stress. If there is a drought, such as a bad day or week, or other forms of stress, we can maintain a healthy state because there is a supply in our reservoirs.

We know that sometimes being a caregiver can be difficult and challenging, and this can drain our reservoirs. If the reservoirs are dry, we can become vulnerable to stresses: there may be some energy or happiness, but only if daily events are going well. The combination of a dry reservoir and a bad day could be problematic and might lead to difficulties, such as an emotional crash, a lost temper, frustration, and so forth.

These workshops aim to teach you different ways of maintaining or replenishing your reservoirs so that you can maintain well-being and do more of what's important in life.

Introducing Values (Active)

Aim: To introduce the concept of values, areas of life that might be important to participants, as well as barriers to values.

To start, ask participants for examples of values, and write them on a whiteboard. You can use the following examples as prompts while encouraging the group participants to share their own ideas:

- Relationships (e.g., to be more loving to your partner)

- Personal growth and health (e.g., maintaining good physical health)

- Work and education (e.g., a job that gives one a sense of satisfaction)

- Leisure (e.g., family activities one enjoys)

Dialogue Example

These workshops are about focusing on what is important to you in life, or your values. Values are our heart's deepest desires regarding how we act in the world and interact with other people. They're what we want to stand for in life, how we want to behave; they are representative of the sort of person we want to be, the qualities we want to develop, and how we want to embody what matters to us.

Participants often identify goals rather than values, so it is important to clarify the difference. Explain that *values* are like directions we want to move in life, whereas *goals* are things that we want to achieve or complete.

Dialogue Example

The difference between getting married and being loving can illustrate the difference between values and goals. If you want to be loving and caring, that's a value—it's ongoing; you want to behave that way for the rest of your life. And in any moment you have a choice: you can act on your value or neglect it. Getting married is a goal. It is something that you can achieve, even if you neglect the value of being loving.

Barriers to Values

Besides introducing the concept of values, it's important to acknowledge and discuss barriers that can interfere with living a valued life. Ask participants about the process of thinking about what is important to them. See if participants notice their mind coming up with barriers (e.g., memories, self-critical thoughts, emotions) that might prevent them from moving in valued directions. Validate that this is what minds do, particularly when we plan to head in a direction that is important.

On a whiteboard write down examples of barriers that people identify. If necessary, provide examples of thoughts (*I can't do this*), emotions (such as anxiety), and physical sensations (such as the heart beating fast). Highlight the distinction between internal (e.g., thoughts, feelings, bodily sensations) and external (e.g., money, time) barriers, and discuss how we have less control over external barriers but can learn to respond differently to internal ones.

Introducing the Passengers on the Bus Metaphor

Aim: To introduce the passengers on the bus metaphor, the central metaphor of the workshop sessions.

It's important to introduce the passengers on the bus metaphor to participants early on.

Passengers on the Bus Metaphor

One way to think about barriers is to think about them as passengers on the bus of life.

Imagine life is like a journey, and you're the driver of your bus. You want to go places and do what's important for you. Over the course of your life, various passengers have boarded your bus. They reflect your thoughts, feelings, and all kinds of inner states. Some of them you like, such as happy memories or positive thoughts, and some you feel neutral about. And then there are passengers that you wish had not boarded the bus; they can be ugly, scary, and nasty.

So, you are driving your bus of life with all sorts of passengers on board. The scary passengers can threaten you and want to be at the front of the bus where you see them. You take this very seriously and stop the bus to struggle and fight with them. You may try to avoid them, distract yourself, or throw them off the bus, but they are your inner states, so you can't get rid of them. However, while the bus is stopped, you're not moving in the direction that's important to you.

You may also try to make deals with the passengers; you'll give in and do what they tell you to do if they agree to keep quiet in the back of the bus. This may feel a little easier than fighting with them, but it means the passengers are in control of the direction your bus is heading.

By fighting and struggling with the passengers or giving in to them, you, the driver, are not in control of your journey of life, and it's likely that you are not heading in a direction that is important to you. But what if, even though these passengers look scary, nasty, and threatening, they can't take control unless you allow them to? There can be different ways to respond to the passengers so that you can head in the direction that is important.

After introducing the metaphor, show the passengers on the bus video, which you can download at http://www.actforpsychosis.com. Explain that the short film animates the story of Tom, his bus of life, and his passengers. Ask participants to listen closely to what his passengers say and observe how he responds to them.

During the animation, pause the video at certain points to briefly discuss what is happening to Tom and his passengers; this will help participants retain information about the story. Useful stopping points include when Tom gives in to his passengers and returns to the Same Old Road, when he decides to fight and struggle with his passengers, or when he witnesses another bus driver respond differently to passengers.

After the video, have people debrief in pairs, discussing what they noticed about the different ways Tom responded to his passengers and what they feel his goals and valued direction may have been.

Automatic Pilot

After participants have had time to discuss the video, introduce the concept of noticing, and highlight the difference between being in contact with the present moment and being on automatic pilot.

Automatic Pilot

A part of what these workshops will be about is helping you become more aware of what is going on inside yourself, including noticing thoughts, feelings, and bodily sensations, as well as outside yourself, including sights and sounds. One way to do this is by practicing being in the present moment.

Does anyone know what "automatic pilot" means? It means doing things without bringing our conscious awareness to them, such as brushing our teeth or driving a car. Automatic pilot isn't necessarily bad, because it would be unhelpful to think about every movement when performing such activities.

Unfortunately, we are often on automatic pilot in many other areas of our life. This means that sometimes we don't think before we respond, or we don't notice what our bodies, emotions, and behaviors are telling us. Learning to purposefully pay attention and notice helps us be more aware of these experiences, and being more aware means we have more freedom to choose how we respond.

We can practice the skill of becoming more aware by noticing where our attention is and learning to deliberately shift its focus. We can do this by focusing on our body, using our breath or five senses to bring us into the present moment. From this place we are able to observe what's going on for us emotionally, physically, and mentally.

Mindfulness Exercise (Aware)

Aim: To introduce the mindfulness of breath and body, and to guide participants through the exercise, allowing time for an inquiry afterward.

Before introducing the first mindfulness exercise, provide participants with some guidance about such noticing exercises. For example, let them know that you will be introducing a brief noticing exercise, in which a facilitator will guide them to notice their breath and body, and that the exercise will last approximately five minutes. Let them know that they can either close their eyes or focus on a spot in front of them during the exercise, if that's more comfortable.

It can be helpful to highlight that there is no right or wrong way of noticing, and that the aim is not to try to change any experiences or pass judgment, but just simply to allow themselves to notice whatever experiences are present.

Mindfulness of Breath and Body Exercise

I invite you to sit in a comfortable yet upright position in your chair, with your feet flat on the floor, arms and legs uncrossed, and hands resting in your lap. [Pause.] Let your eyes gently close, or fix them on a point in front of you. [Pause five seconds.]

Begin by gently bringing your attention to noticing your body. Start by directing your attention to your feet [pause]; notice the parts of your feet that are in contact with the ground. [Pause five seconds.] Notice the sensation of your shoes or socks on your feet. [Pause five seconds.] Then, bring your attention to noticing the sensation of sitting in the chair. [Pause.] See if you can notice the sense of your weight on the chair. [Pause five seconds.] Maybe notice parts of your body that are in contact with the chair [pause], and the parts of your body that don't contact the chair. [Pause five seconds.] If you drift off into your thoughts, simply acknowledge where your mind went and bring it back to noticing the sensation of sitting in the chair. [Pause five seconds.]

From time to time, you may notice that your attention has wandered off as you get caught up in your thoughts or other kinds of sensations. This is quite normal; it happens to everyone, and it may happen repeatedly. Each time you notice your mind wandering, take a split second to notice where it took you and gently bring your awareness back to noticing your body and the sense of your weight on the chair. [Pause five seconds.]

Next, direct your awareness to your breath. [Pause five seconds.] See if you can notice the sensation of breathing in [pause] and out [pause five seconds], allowing your stomach to expand, and your chest to gently rise and fall. [Pause five seconds.] Become aware of your breath, flowing in and out, and of your body. Simply notice the natural flow of the breath, without changing or modifying it in any way. [Pause five seconds.]

Take a few slow, deep breaths. Notice the sensation of air filling your lungs as you breathe in and then deflating as you breathe out. [Pause five seconds.] You may notice the sensation of cool air around your nostrils as you inhale [pause], and the warm air as you exhale. [Pause five seconds.]

As you do this exercise, the feelings and sensations in your body may change. You may notice pleasant feelings or sensations, such as relaxation, calmness, or peacefulness. [Pause.] You may notice unpleasant feelings, such as boredom, frustration, or anxiety. [Pause.] Whatever feelings, urges, or sensations arise, whether pleasant or unpleasant, gently acknowledge their presence and let them be. Allow them to come and go, and keep your attention on your breath and the sensation of sitting in the chair. [Pause five seconds.]

Lastly, bring your attention back to noticing your breathing. [Pause five to ten seconds.] Notice again the steady rhythm of your breath that is with you all the time. [Pause five to ten seconds.] When you are ready, bring your attention back to the room. Open your eyes if they are closed. Notice what you can see [pause], and notice what you can hear. [Pause.] Push your feet into the ground and stretch and notice yourself stretching. Welcome back.

After completing the exercise, invite observations from participants. Inquire about what they noticed, and invite curiosity about the experience. Focus on drawing out differences between this experience and automatic-pilot experiences.

Highlight that mindfulness can be applied to any activity, from mundane, boring tasks done every day to those that are important. Note that being mindful of daily activities allows us to experience them and be truly alive in the moment.

Dialogue Example

What did people notice when doing that exercise? Were you able to notice your body and the sensation of sitting in the chair? Did you notice your breath? Were you aware of your mind wandering off during the exercise? Were you able to bring your attention back to noticing your body and breath?

We suggest that facilitators take their time in the inquiry, as this is often a key place for learning. Work to ensure that any feedback is validated and reinforced. Model a stance of equal curiosity toward all points raised by participants. Emphasize any learning that happened, and try not to problem solve or provide expert answers or solutions.

Closing the Session

Aim: To bring the group session to a close, to encourage participants to provide feedback on their experience of the session, and to encourage workshop attendance.

Come back together as a large group and ask for feedback about the workshop session. Ask participants how they generally found the session, and what they found most memorable. Reinforce the importance of attending next week's session.

To prompt feedback, consider writing the following on a whiteboard:

- How did you find the session to be today?

- What did you notice?

- What did you find helpful or unhelpful, or both?

- What was the most memorable thing from today's workshop?

If short on time, you could ask for "popcorn feedback": ask everyone to say one or two words to sum up what they found most memorable from the day's session.

SESSION 1

Introducing Noticing, Values, and Committed Action

Session 1 is intended to introduce the participants—whether clients or caregivers—to the series of workshop sessions, as well as the concepts of noticing, values, and barriers to values. Facilitators will introduce the idea of automatic pilot and lead the group through the mindfulness of breath and body and noticing exercises. The facilitator will then introduce committed actions and SMART goals, after which participants will engage in small group exercises and complete a committed action worksheet. The session closes with a discussion of dates for future workshops. The following session outline suggests an order for the topics and time frames. As always, the times given for each segment are approximate.

Certain elements of the taster session are covered in session 1 because some participants may not have attended the taster session, and these are important elements to discuss. Covering them again can act as a refresher of skills and an extended discussion for those who attended the taster session.

Timeline

Welcome and introduction	10 minutes
Noticing exercise (aware)	20 minutes
Introducing values (active)	30 minutes
Introducing the passengers on the bus metaphor	35 minutes
Noticing exercise (aware)	5 minutes
Setting committed actions (active)	15 minutes
Closing the session	5 minutes

Materials You'll Need

- Whiteboard
- Paper and pens
- Marker pens
- Folders
- Refreshments
- Mindfulness CDs or USB sticks
- Values worksheets
- Passengers on the bus worksheets
- Committed action worksheets
- Developing aware skills worksheets

Welcome and Introduction

Aim: To make participants feel welcome and to highlight the purpose of the workshop sessions by working through key points on the whiteboard.

Welcome participants to session 1 (of 4) of the ACT for recovery workshop. Explain that the workshop sessions will run for approximately two hours, with a short break halfway through. Introduce housekeeping issues (e.g., fire escapes, bathrooms). Facilitators should introduce themselves and their roles and write their names on a name badge. Ask participants to also wear name badges. Highlight the purposes of the workshop sessions by working through the key points on a whiteboard:

- Developing life direction
- Increasing awareness of obstacles
- Learning the skills of open, aware, and active in order to respond more effectively to obstacles
- Connecting with each other and having fun

Dialogue Example

Here are some of the key points for this series of workshops. We'll be exploring each of these areas session by session.

Ground Rules

After discussing the key points, it's a good idea to agree on ground rules for the workshop sessions. Facilitators should provide initial ideas for ground rules on a whiteboard and then ask the group to generate others, adding to the whiteboard those the group agrees upon. It's a good idea to display the ground rules during each session, in case participants need to be reminded of them. Here are some possibilities for initial rules:

- Respect what other people notice.
- Keep what is said in the group within the group.
- Listen to other people.
- Be punctual and attend the sessions.
- Mobile phones should be silent.
- Any others?

Dialogue Example

We find it useful in workshops to think of ground rules together to make sure that people feel safe enough to share their experiences. What would we need to agree to so that you feel this is a safe space to talk?

Warm-Up Exercise

After brainstorming ground rules, help participants get warmed up for the workshop session with a brief exercise. Invite the participants to discuss with the person next to them three things they like to do. Facilitators can give examples (e.g., I like to travel, I like to go to the movies). Afterward, draw links between the examples given and values. It can be helpful to give participants a pen and paper to write down what their partner has told them. When addressing the larger group, this can help them remember what the person said.

Dialogue Example

To get us started, we'd like to invite you to do a short warm-up exercise. With the person next to you, discuss three things that you both like to do. One thing I like to do is watch movies. Now, spend a few minutes discussing what you like doing. Then we'll come back to the larger group and we'll ask you to introduce your partner and tell the group one of the three things he or she likes to do.

Reservoir Metaphor (Caregiver Workshops)

At this point in sessions for caregivers, it's time to introduce the reservoir metaphor as a way of identifying how important it is for them to maintain their own well-being, and how the workshops may be useful for this. If this is a session for clients, skip this metaphor.

The Reservoir Metaphor

We all have "emotional reservoirs" of different types. Some supply energy, others supply health or well-being. When the reservoirs are full, we can maintain our energy or well-being, even in times of stress. If there is a drought, such as a bad day or week, or other forms of stress, we can maintain a healthy state because there is a supply in our reservoirs.

We know that sometimes being a caregiver can be difficult and challenging, and this can drain our reservoirs. If the reservoirs are dry, we can become vulnerable to stresses: there may be some energy or happiness, but only if daily events are going well. The combination of a dry reservoir and a bad day could be problematic and might lead to difficulties, such as an emotional crash, a lost temper, frustration, and so forth.

These workshops aim to teach you different ways of maintaining or replenishing your reservoirs so that you can maintain well-being and do more of what's important in life.

Automatic Pilot

After the warm-up exercise, introduce the concept of noticing, and highlight the difference between being in contact with the present moment and being on automatic pilot.

Automatic Pilot

A part of what these workshops will be about is helping you to become more aware of what is going on inside yourself, including noticing thoughts, feelings, and bodily sensations, as well as outside yourself, including sights and sounds. One way to develop the skill of noticing is by practicing being in the present moment.

Does anyone know what "automatic pilot" means? It means doing things without bringing our conscious awareness to them, such as brushing our teeth or driving a car. Automatic pilot isn't necessarily bad, because it would be unhelpful to think about every movement when performing such activities.

Unfortunately, we are often on automatic pilot in many other areas of our life. This means that sometimes we don't think before we respond, or we don't listen to what our bodies, emotions, and behaviors are telling us. Learning to purposefully pay attention helps us to be more aware of these experiences, and being more aware means we have more freedom to choose how we respond.

We can practice the skill of becoming more aware by noticing where our attention is and learning to deliberately shift its focus. We can do this by focusing on our body, using our breath or five senses to bring us into the present moment. From this place we are able to observe what's going on for us emotionally, physically, and mentally.

Noticing Exercise (Aware)

Aim: To introduce the mindfulness of breath and body, and to guide participants through a noticing exercise, allowing time for an inquiry afterward.

Before introducing the first mindfulness exercise, provide participants with some guidance about such noticing exercises. For example, let them know that you will be introducing a brief noticing exercise, in which a facilitator will guide them to notice their breath and body, and that the exercise will last approximately five minutes. Let them know that during the exercise they can either close their eyes or focus on a spot in front of them, if that's more comfortable.

It can be helpful to highlight that there is no right or wrong way of noticing, and that the aim is not to try to change any experiences or pass judgment, rather it's to just simply allow themselves to notice whatever experiences are present.

Mindfulness of Breath and Body Exercise

I invite you to sit in a comfortable yet upright position in your chair, with your feet flat on the floor, arms and legs uncrossed, and hands resting in your lap. [Pause.] Let your eyes gently close, or fix them on a point in front of you. [Pause five seconds.]

Begin by gently bringing your attention to noticing your body. Start by directing your attention to your feet [pause]; notice the parts of your feet that are in contact with the ground. [Pause five seconds.] Notice the sensation of your shoes or socks on your feet. [Pause five seconds.] Then, bring your attention to noticing the sensation of sitting in the chair. [Pause.] See if you can notice the sense of your weight on the chair. [Pause five seconds.] Maybe notice parts of your body that are in contact with the chair [pause], and the parts of your body that don't contact the chair. [Pause five seconds.] If you drift off into your thoughts, simply acknowledge where your mind went and bring it back to noticing the sensation of sitting in the chair. [Pause five seconds.]

From time to time, you may notice that your attention has wandered off as you get caught up in your thoughts or other kinds of sensations. This is quite normal; it happens to everyone, and it may happen repeatedly. Each time you notice your mind wandering, take a split second to notice where it took you and gently bring your awareness back to noticing your body and the sense of your weight on the chair. [Pause five seconds.]

Next, direct your awareness to your breath. [Pause five seconds.] See if you can notice the sensation of breathing in [pause] and out [pause five seconds], allowing your stomach to expand, and your chest to gently rise and fall. [Pause five seconds.] Become aware of your breath, flowing in and out, and of your body. Simply notice the natural flow of the breath, without changing or modifying it in any way. [Pause five seconds.]

Take a few slow, deep breaths. Notice the sensation of air filling your lungs as you breathe in and then deflating as you breathe out. [Pause five seconds.] You may notice the sensation of cool air around your nostrils as you inhale [pause], and the warm air as you exhale. [Pause five seconds.]

As you do this exercise, the feelings and sensations in your body may change. You may notice pleasant feelings or sensations, such as relaxation, calmness, or peacefulness. [Pause.] You may notice unpleasant feelings, such as boredom, frustration, or anxiety. [Pause.] Whatever feelings, urges, or sensations arise, whether pleasant or unpleasant, gently acknowledge their presence and let them be. Allow them to come and go, and keep your attention on your breath and the sensation of sitting in the chair. [Pause five seconds.]

Lastly, bring your attention back to noticing your breathing. [Pause five to ten seconds.] Notice again the steady rhythm of your breath that is with you all the time. [Pause five to ten seconds.] When you are ready, bring your attention back to the room. Open your eyes if they are closed. Notice what you can see [pause], and notice what you can hear. [Pause.] Push your feet into the ground and stretch and notice yourself stretching. Welcome back.

After completing the exercise, invite observations from participants. Inquire about what they noticed, and invite curiosity about the experience. Focus on drawing out differences between this experience and automatic-pilot experiences.

Highlight that mindfulness can be applied to any activity, from mundane, boring tasks done every day to those that are more important. Note that being mindful of daily activities allows us to experience them and be truly alive in the moment.

Dialogue Example

What did people notice when doing that exercise? Were you able to notice your body and the sensation of sitting in the chair? Did you notice your breath? Were you aware of your mind wandering off during the exercise? Were you able to bring your attention back to noticing your body and breath?

We suggest that facilitators take their time in the inquiry, as this is often a key place for learning. Work to ensure that any feedback is validated and reinforced. Model a stance of equal curiosity toward all points raised by participants. Emphasize any learning that happened, and try not to problem solve or provide expert answers or solutions.

Introducing Values (Active)

Aim: To introduce the concept of values, areas of life that might be important to participants, as well as barriers to values.

To start, ask participants for examples of values, and write them on a whiteboard. You can use the following examples as prompts while encouraging the group participants to share their own ideas:

- Relationships (e.g., to be more loving to your partner)

- Personal growth and health (e.g., maintaining good physical health)
- Work and education (e.g., a job that gives one a sense of satisfaction)
- Leisure (e.g., family activities one enjoys)

Dialogue Example

These workshops are about focusing on what is important to you in life, or your values. Values are our heart's deepest desires regarding how we act in the world and interact with other people. They're what we want to stand for in life, how we want to behave; they are representative of the sort of person we want to be, the qualities we want to develop, and how we want to embody what matters to us.

Values Worksheets

After introducing values as a concept, have participants complete values worksheets. These should encourage them to identify valued directions they may want to move in during the workshop sessions. At this point, clarify that values—chosen life directions and choices—are not feelings, successful outcomes, or achievements, nor are they always easy!

Break into small groups (one facilitator to lead each group) and ask participants to take a few minutes to think about a valued direction they may want to move in during the workshop sessions. See if they can picture themselves moving in this direction. In the interest of time, ask participants to complete just one part of the values worksheet. This exercise is to familiarize them with the concept. They can complete the rest of the worksheet over the coming weeks or as homework. Facilitators can assist participants to identify their values and complete the worksheet. If you notice people identifying goals, try to explore the value behind the goal. For example, you could ask, "What would it mean to you if you achieved this, and why is that important?"

Barriers to Values

See if participants noticed their mind coming up with barriers (e.g., memories, self-critical thoughts, emotions) that might prevent them from moving in valued directions. Validate that this is what minds do, particularly when we plan to head in a direction that is important.

On a whiteboard write down examples of barriers that people identify. If necessary, provide examples of thoughts (*I can't do this*), emotions (such as anxiety), and physical sensations (such as the heart beating fast). Highlight the distinction between internal (e.g., thoughts, feelings, bodily sensations) and external (e.g., money, time) barriers, and discuss how we have less control over external barriers but can learn to respond differently to internal ones.

Introducing the Passengers on the Bus Metaphor

Aim: To introduce the passengers on the bus metaphor, the central metaphor of the workshop sessions.

Passengers on the Bus Metaphor

One way to think about barriers is to think about them as passengers on the bus of life.

Imagine life is like a journey, and you're the driver of your bus. You want to go places and do what's important for you. Over the course of your life, various passengers have boarded your bus. They reflect your thoughts, feelings, and all kinds of inner states. Some of them you like, such as happy memories or positive thoughts, and some you feel neutral about. And then there are passengers that you wish had not boarded the bus; they can be ugly, scary, and nasty.

So, you are driving your bus of life with all sorts of passengers on board. The scary passengers can threaten you and want to be at the front of the bus where you see them. You take this very seriously and stop the bus to struggle and fight with them. You may try to avoid them, distract yourself, or throw them off the bus, but they are your inner states, so you can't get rid of them. However, while the bus is stopped, you're not moving in the direction that's important to you.

You may also try to make deals with the passengers; you'll give in and do what they tell you to do if they agree to keep quiet in the back of the bus. This may feel a little easier than fighting with them, but it means the passengers are in control of the direction your bus is heading.

By fighting and struggling with the passengers or giving in to them, you, the driver, are not in control of your journey of life, and it's likely that you are not heading in a direction that is important to you. But what if, even though these passengers look scary, nasty, and threatening, they can't take control unless you allow them to? There can be different ways to respond to the passengers so that you can head in the direction that is important.

After introducing the metaphor, show the passengers on the bus video, which you can download at http://www.actforpsychosis.com. Explain that the short film animates the story of Tom, his bus of life, and his passengers. Ask participants to listen closely to what his passengers say and how he responds to them.

During the animation, pause the video at certain points to briefly discuss what is happening to Tom and his passengers; this will help participants retain information about the story. Useful stopping points include when Tom gives in to his passengers and returns to the Same Old Road, when he decides to fight and struggle with his passengers, or when he witnesses a different bus driver respond differently to passengers.

After the video, have people debrief in pairs, discussing what they noticed about the different ways Tom responded to his passengers and what they feel his goals and valued direction may have been.

Once you've finished discussing the content of the video, have participants break into small groups to complete the passengers on the bus worksheet. Have them highlight a value from their values worksheet and then identify the passengers that might prevent them from moving toward or acting on this value. Ask them to identify how they might respond to these passengers (e.g., fight and struggle, give in). Facilitators can provide examples to help participants complete the worksheet.

Dialogue Example

One thing that is important to me is maintaining my physical health. Some of the passengers that show up and get in the way of me moving in this direction are "feeling tired," "forgetting," and an inner voice that says "Do it another day."

While completing the worksheet, encourage participants to focus on internal barriers (e.g., thoughts, feelings, memories) rather than external ones (e.g., money, time, other people). If need be, refer back to the whiteboard examples of barriers (e.g., emotions, such as feeling too depressed; thoughts, such as *What's the point?* or *Others won't notice*). And finally, ask for feedback on the process of completing the worksheet and identifying passengers.

Some participants may struggle to identify passengers. Facilitators can provide support by helping them identify what is getting in the way of moving toward what they have identified as important. Also, remind participants that we will be returning to the worksheets throughout the workshop, so they can add to the worksheets whenever they notice more passengers.

Noticing Exercise (Aware)

Aim: To guide participants through the mindful stretch exercise and to debrief afterward.

Introduce this short noticing exercise as a way for participants to step out of automatic mode and reconnect with the present moment. Before commencing, stress that it is important for them to be aware of their body and its limitations. For each of the stretches you'll describe, they should just be aware of what their body is telling them. Recommend that they approach the practice gently and with curiosity, and, as best they can, they should notice if they are competing with someone else or with their own body. Highlight the importance of bringing attention to the experience in the present moment, listening to the limits of your body, and respecting those limits, not pushing through them. Emphasize that they should allow their body to be as it is, with all the strengths and limitations that it has right now. Feel free to invite participants to take their shoes off, if that feels comfortable to them, and remind them that they can keep their eyes open during the exercise.

Mindful Stretch Exercise

Begin by standing with your feet flat on the ground, hip-width apart. [Pause.] Notice how it feels to stand here [pause], noticing the sensations of the ground beneath your feet and the sensations in your body right now. Allow your shoulders to relax as best you can, and be present in your body. [Pause.] Start to bring your awareness to your breath and your stomach, being here, standing here, and breathing. [Pause five seconds.]

If you can, slowly begin to move your arms out to the side of your body. Gently allow your arms to move upward, bringing awareness to the environment around your arms, noticing whatever sensations are here as your arms rise. [Pause.] And gently bring the arms upward, slowly and mindfully until they're right up over your head, reaching for the sky. [Pause.]

Now, very gently, begin to move your arms over to the right so your body is slightly bending over. You might notice your hips moving slightly out to the left. [Pause.] Just notice whatever sensations you experience during this stretch. And, when you feel ready, move your arms back to the center.

Next, allow your arms to move over to the left side. Your hips may move over to the right and your body very gently bends to the left. Just notice the sensations of the stretch. Then, very slowly, mindfully come back up to the center, and gently lower your arms to your sides. Notice whatever sensations that are here; notice any tendency for the arms to rush back to the side of your body. [Pause five seconds.]

When your arms reach your sides, just notice how your body is feeling right now. Notice any sensations of having done this stretch and being present, standing here with your feet on the ground, breathing and being aware of your breath. [Pause five seconds.]

Now, allow your hands to rest on your hips so your elbows are out to the sides. Settle into this posture, and, with your hips and feet still facing forward, very gently turn your upper body to the right. Keep your feet and hips facing forward, your upper body and shoulders moving to the right, just as far as they'll go. Not pushing anything, just gently twisting your body as far as it wants to be twisted right now. Then, gently, mindfully, come back to the center.

And now, gently twist your body to the left. Your feet steady on the ground, your hips facing forward, your shoulders and your upper body gently turned to the left as far as they will go. Then, gently coming back to the center, noticing the sensations of the stretch. Now, allow your arms to fall to the side of your body. [Pause five seconds.]

Slowly move your head toward your right shoulder, gently stretching your neck just as far as it wants to go, noticing the sensation. Now, slowly come back to the center. Then, gently move your head to your left shoulder, mindfully stretching. Just noticing how your body feels right now. Then, bring your head back to the center and settle into this posture. [Pause five seconds.]

Come back to standing with your feet flat on the floor, your arms resting by your sides, your shoulders back, your head straight, just resting here in this pose. Bring your awareness to your stomach and the rise and fall as you breathe in, and as you breathe out. Standing here in awareness, breathing, noticing how your body feels having done these stretches. [Pause.]

And, as this period of practice comes to an end, just rest here, and when you move away from this posture, see if you can bring mindfulness to your body as you move on into the day.

After completing the exercise, invite observations from participants. Ask about what they noticed, and invite curiosity about the experience.

Dialogue Example

What did people notice while doing this exercise? Were you able to notice your body and the sensation of different stretches? Did you notice any difference before and after each stretch? Were people aware of their mind wandering off during the exercise? Were you able to bring your attention back to noticing your body and the different stretches?

Setting Committed Actions

Aim: To set committed actions to be completed during the week.

To start this portion of the session, write the following questions and guidelines on a whiteboard:

- Think of one action you could take that would move you toward a value.
- What passengers might get in the way as you try to take this action?
- How might you respond to these passengers?
- Try to practice a noticing exercise during the following week.

Then have participants break into small groups, with one facilitator for each group. Ask participants to complete a committed action worksheet in order to identify one values-based action they can take during the next week that might move them toward their values. Ask that they try and set a SMART goal:

- **S**pecific
- **M**easurable
- **A**chievable
- **R**ealistic
- **T**ime-oriented

Within the small groups, ask participants if they would be willing to tell the others what they plan to do over the next week, and reinforce anything they say that suggests a willingness to share their commitments with others. Also, determine if participants would like one of the facilitators to contact them for a short five-minute phone call between sessions to discuss how their committed actions are going. Make it clear that the phone calls are not designed as checkups to determine whether the person has completed the action, rather they serve as reminders of the aspects of the committed-action process, such as mindful noticing and willingness. Highlight that you are interested in what participants notice when working toward their committed actions, particularly any passengers that might show up and how they respond to them. Emphasize that if they achieve their committed actions, that is an added bonus to the process.

Dialogue Example

Think about the important valued direction you identified earlier in the session. Can you think of one action you could do over the next week that would reflect that this is something important? Keep in mind that this is an opportunity to practice mindful noticing of passengers and your responses to them. If you complete the action, that's icing on the cake.

One thing that is important to me is maintaining my physical health, and a goal linked to this is to go to the gym this week. My SMART action to move me closer to this goal is to go the gym twice this week, as I feel this is both achievable and realistic. To make sure my goals are time oriented, I will go on Tuesday and Saturday this week for at least thirty minutes (measurable). I will note these visits in my diary so I don't forget them. I will also pack my bag so I am ready to attend the gym when I finish work. Maintaining my physical health is important to me, so I'm going to write this in the "values connected with my action" section. Some of the passengers who may show up and get in the way of me moving toward this value are "feeling too tired," "forgetting," and "feeling self-conscious."

Before breaking up the small groups, ask participants to complete the developing aware skills worksheet, and see if they would be willing to practice the mindfulness of breath and body exercise at least three times over the next week.

Closing the Session

Aim: To bring the group session to a close and encourage participants to offer feedback about their experiences of the session.

Come back together as a large group and ask for feedback about the workshop session. Ask participants how they generally found the session, and what they found most memorable. Reinforce the importance of attending next week's session.

To prompt feedback, consider writing the following on a whiteboard:

- How did you find the session to be today?
- What did you notice?
- What did you find helpful or unhelpful, or both?
- What was the most memorable thing from today's workshop?

If short on time, you could ask for "popcorn feedback": ask everyone to say one or two words to sum up what they found most memorable from the day's session.

SESSION 2

Workability as an Alternative

The main purpose of session 2 is to introduce the participants—whether clients or caregivers—to the concept of openness as an alternative to struggling, and to practice the passengers on the bus metaphor. First, facilitators and participants will discuss the purpose of the workshop and what happened in the last session before doing a warm-up exercise. A facilitator will lead the group through the mindful eating exercise, followed by an inquiry debrief. The group will then review the passengers on the bus metaphor before breaking into small groups to review their committed actions. Then they will watch a video and discuss its relation to the passengers on the bus metaphor. A facilitator will introduce and lead the group through the willingness exercise (pushing against the folder), followed by a debrief. The group will then act out the passengers on the bus metaphor with a focus on how one responds to the various passengers. Afterward, a facilitator will lead the group through the three-minute breathing space exercise, after which participants will break into small groups and complete committed action worksheets. The session closes with a facilitator asking for feedback on today's session and encouraging participants to attend the next session. The following session outline suggests an order for the topics and time frames. As always, the times given for each segment are approximate.

Timeline

Welcome and introduction	10 minutes
Noticing exercise (aware)	15 minutes
Passengers on the bus review	5 minutes
Committed action review	10 minutes
Video vignette	20 minutes
Willingness exercise (open)	10 minutes
Acting out the passengers on the bus exercise (open)	25 minutes
Noticing exercise (aware)	5 minutes
Committed action (active)	10 minutes
Closing the session	5 minutes

Materials You'll Need

- Whiteboard
- Projector and speakers
- Paper and pens
- Marker pens
- Refreshments
- Committed action worksheets
- Folders (for willingness exercise)
- Developing Aware Skills Worksheet

Additional Equipment for This Session

- A soft ball
- Sticky notes
- Clementines for the mindful eating exercise (one for each participant and facilitator)

Welcome and Introduction

Aim: To welcome participants to session 2 (of 4) of the ACT for recovery workshop.

Remind people that the workshop will run for approximately two hours with a short break halfway through. If required, take care of housekeeping issues (e.g., location of fire escapes, bathrooms). Ask people again to wear name badges. As a refresher, review the purpose of the workshops by reading through the following points on the whiteboard:

- Developing life direction
- Increasing awareness of obstacles
- Learning the skills of open, aware, and active in order to respond more effectively to obstacles
- Connecting with each other and having fun

Dialogue Example

Just to remind you, here are some of the key points for this series of workshops. We'll be exploring each of these areas week by week.

After reviewing the purposes of the workshop, it's helpful to recap what happened in session 1 by writing out points on the whiteboard:

- The mindful skill of noticing
- Thinking about what's important in life (values)
- What gets in the way of moving toward values
- The passengers on the bus metaphor

Dialogue Example

Here are some of the main topics we talked about last week. First, we introduced the idea of mindful noticing. Then we talked about things that are important in life. Lastly, we introduced the passengers on the bus metaphor and discussed what passengers get in the way of leading a meaningful life.

After the review, help participants warm up for the session with a brief exercise. Invite everyone to stand up, and ask them what they would take to a desert island and why. Facilitators can start the exercise by giving examples ("I would take pictures of my family members to remind me of how important they are."). Afterward, draw links between participants' examples and how they reflect what is important to them.

Dialogue Example

To get us started, we'd like to invite you to do a short warm-up exercise. The person holding the ball briefly says what she would take to a desert island and why and then passes the ball to another person, who says what he'd take before passing the ball on, and so on until we've all had a turn.

Noticing Exercise (Aware)

Aim: To introduce and guide people through the noticing exercise, leaving enough time to carry out an inquiry afterward.

Before beginning the exercise, make sure each participant has a clementine (or similar fruit) in hand. When facilitating this exercise, it's helpful to keep an eye on how quickly participants peel their clementine and to only move on when everyone is at the same point.

Dialogue Example

Now, we are going to spend a few minutes getting present and practicing being aware of an object, in this case a clementine.

Mindful Eating Exercise

We spend a lot of our lives not really being present in the here and now. Life can be busy and our minds can be easily distracted by our passengers. So now we are going to spend a few minutes focusing on the present by spending time noticing an object.

I'd like you to take the object you've been given and examine it. [Pause.]

Observe it with curiosity, as if you've never seen an object like this before. [Pause.]

Study its shape, its contours. [Pause five seconds.]

Notice its colors. Are there many different shades to it? [Pause five seconds.]

Notice the weight of it in your hand [pause], and the feel of it against your skin. [Pause.]

Run your fingers over the object and notice the way that the skin feels. [Pause.]

Raise it to your nose and smell it; really notice the aroma. [Pause.]

Break open the skin and notice what is inside. [Pause five seconds.]

Raise it to your nose again and see if there is a change in the aroma. [Pause.]

Notice the texture on the inside of the object. [Pause.]

Take out one segment of the object; hold it in your hand. [Pause.]

Feel the object between your fingers. [Pause.]

Take a moment to really study it. [Pause.]

Gently squeeze it and notice its texture. [Pause.]

Then, if you are willing, gently place the segment in your mouth. Don't chew it—just roll it around in your mouth. [Pause five seconds.]

Notice what's happening in your mouth; notice the salivation. [Pause.]

Notice the urge to bite. [Pause.]

When you are ready, bite into the object. Notice how it tastes. Notice the texture. [Pause five seconds.]

Slowly chew the object, and notice the sensations as you swallow it. [Pause.]

[End by linking to values and purpose.] Even with a small object like this clementine, we can notice more by focusing on the present moment. Notice your experience of this object by being with it in this particular way. And now notice being here in the room, your purpose for coming here today, and the passengers that you carry with you while doing this.

After completing the exercise, invite observations from participants. Ask about what they noticed and invite curiosity about the experience. Focus on drawing out differences between this experience and automatic-pilot experiences.

Dialogue Example

What did people notice when doing this exercise? Did people notice more flavor and taste for this segment of clementine? Is this how you normally eat a clementine? In what ways is it different? Do you sometimes just eat quickly and automatically without noticing the flavors and sensations?

Consider that this type of noticing can be applied to any activity you engage in, from mundane, boring tasks you do every day to those that are more important. Being mindful of daily activities allows us to experience them and be truly alive in the moment.

Draw out the ways participants responded automatically in the exercise (for example, chewing and swallowing quickly), noting how easy this kind of behavior is. Note how this contrasts to the deliberate skill being practiced in the exercise and how this skill may be applicable to other areas of life.

Passengers on the Bus Review

Aim: To remind people about the key elements of the passengers on the bus video shown in session 1, including valued directions, the role of passengers, and their responses to passengers. Remember to ask the group what they remember of the metaphor first before explaining it.

Dialogue Example: General

This metaphor is about the directions we want to go—our values—and the passengers that are on our bus who come along for the ride.

Dialogue Example: Clarifying Passengers

Passengers can be memories, thoughts, feelings, and sensations that can act as barriers to heading in a valued direction. Examples of how we might deal with barriers can be trying to struggle and push the experiences away or giving in to the passengers and allowing them to control the direction of your bus.

Keep in mind that not all passengers are scary or threatening, but they can still prevent us from taking valued actions if we get caught up with them. For example, we might pull over to the side of the road as we get wrapped up in pleasant memories and remembering how life used to be. Or we might get overly focused on a nice feeling, to the exclusion of everything else.

Dialogue Example: Clarifying Valued Directions

Our values are like our chosen life directions or how we "choose" to steer our bus. When we take our hands off the steering wheel in order to deal with these passengers, we are no longer driving the bus or taking valued action.

Sometimes we can easily get caught up with criticizing ourselves for not heading in directions that we "should" be going; for being disappointed by failure; for struggling with the feelings, such as anxiety, that come from moving in valued directions. These can all be additional passengers on our bus that are important to be aware of. The aim is to be able to bring our passengers along for the ride, while noticing the automatic, unhelpful responses toward our passengers that we can get pulled into.

Committed Action Review

Aim: To review the committed action exercise participants completed at the end of the previous session.

On the whiteboard write the following:

- Think of the value you identified and the action linked to this value.

- Did you notice any passengers show up in relation to this action?

- What was your experience of the mindfulness practice?

Then break into small groups with one facilitator to lead each group. Facilitators should review the committed action exercise with each participant and encourage them to either describe what passengers they observed or what they noticed about the process.

Dialogue Example

Toward the end of the previous session, we invited you to try to do something that was important to you, something that you valued. Did anyone have a go at this? What sorts of things did you notice?

How did the mindfulness practice go? Were you able to fit the practice into your usual routines? What did you notice?

When reviewing the committed action exercise, it's useful to keep in mind these points of discussion and style:

- Early in the review process, participants usually offer information regarding content rather than process (for example, describing in detail what they did, rather than reflecting on what they noticed). It's useful to validate this and then draw them into the process of acting on values and noticing obstacles and commonalities between peoples' experiences.

- Highlight any increased awareness of passengers and how people have responded to them.

- Highlight that the main aim is for people to think about taking steps in a valued direction, and that it is a bonus if they are able to do so, but that the main point is to notice the process and what passengers showed up.

- In general, validate feelings but try not to get caught up in problem solving or judgments about experiences. Reinforce noticing and any actions people have taken to move in valued directions. Even spending time thinking about taking action may be a functional improvement, if the participant tends to avoid doing this.

- Validate that some participants may have attended the session even though they didn't feel motivated to do so; perhaps this lack of motivation is another passenger (for example, no fuel in the bus).

- Highlight qualities of committed action: "You can still carry out a valued action, but you can't control the outcome: Is there still value in acting on what is important or meaningful even if it doesn't work out the way you want it to?"

- If participants bring up wanting to feel or stop feeling a certain way (for example, "I want to stop feeling depressed"), suggest that these are "dead person goals," anything a corpse can do better than a live human. For example, a dead person will never feel depressed, never use drugs, and so on. Ask them, "If you weren't feeling depressed, what would you be doing differently in your life?"

- Orient participants to the idea of finding satisfaction in doing all they can: "Our mind can make taking action tricky as it compares, evaluates, and judges. We start from where we start, rather than where our minds say we 'should' be starting from."

- Reinforce all efforts of taking valued action *and* noticing barriers, saying, for example, "There might be lots of things we value and want to pursue. Thinking about doing something is a start, but then barriers and passengers often show up and can get in our way."

Video Vignette

Aim: To watch the video vignette of Paul (for client workshops) or George (for caregiver workshops) and discuss how it's related to the passengers on the bus metaphor.

Before playing the video, on a flip chart write prompts for what participants should watch for as the video plays:

- What passengers are on Paul's/George's bus?
- How does Paul/George respond to his passengers?
- What do you think is important to Paul/George?

Provide participants with paper and pens and ask them to look out for the areas noted above (passengers, responses to passengers, and values). Clarify that the group will then discuss these after the video.

Dialogue Example

To think a little bit more about passengers and buses, we're going to show a short video of someone acting out a made-up story. [Make sure this is clear.] In the video you will see Paul [George], who has been struggling with his passengers. When you watch the video, see if you can spot his passengers, how he responds to them, and also what is important to him.

Review Examples of Paul's Passengers (Client Workshops)

On the whiteboard write the following:

- What passengers are on Paul's bus?
- How did he respond to the passengers?
- What things (values) do you think are important to Paul?

Then ask participants to describe the things—related to the three headings—they noticed on the video, and write their answers on the flip chart. The following examples can be used to prompt the participants.

Paul's Passengers	Paul's Responses to Passengers	Paul's Values
• Difficulty concentrating • Worry • Frustration • Becoming upset • Paranoia (clicking noise on the phone) • "People are watching/recording me." • "I'm unsafe." • Sleep difficulties • "I'm a burden." • Worry: "People are poisoning my food" and "I'm going crazy." • Anxiety	• Working harder, longer hours at work • Taking work home • Challenging others in the office • Talking about the issues • Seeking reassurance • Not sleeping • Not eating • Avoiding situations that make him anxious • Stop seeing friends	• Working hard and enjoying his job • Mutual respect in his relationship with his parents • Having a loving relationship • Supportive friendships

Dialogue Example

Can you relate to any bit of this story? For example, the relief, avoidance, or lack of valued direction? Or do you know anyone who has had experiences like Paul?

What do you notice in terms of the cost to Paul as he responds to his passengers? Does this impact his ability to move toward his values?

We would like to suggest an alternative way to respond to passengers that we don't see Paul using very much. We call this response "openness." An open response is one that eases the struggle and allows for one to continue with values-based actions, while also bringing passengers along for the ride. Let's practice this.

Review Examples of George's Passengers (Caregivers Workshops)

On the whiteboard write the following:

- What passengers are on George's bus?
- How did he respond to the passengers?
- What things (values) do you think are important to George?

Then ask participants to describe the things—related to the three headings—they noticed on the video, and write their answers on the flip chart. The following examples can be used to prompt the participants.

George's Passengers	George's Responses to Passengers	George's Values
• "I passed on the illness through my genes." • "I'm not supported." • Guilt (toward Paul; guilt about colleagues covering his work) • "I'm a bad parent and hopeless father." • Resentment toward Paul	• Arguing with wife • Doing more for Paul to overcompensate • Giving up caring for Paul • Putting Paul's needs in front of his own • Taking time off work • Missing exercise • Stopping seeing friends • Drinking alcohol • Running away from issues	• Caring for his son • Supporting his children • Working hard, to the best of his ability • Having respectful relationships and friendships

Dialogue Example

Can you relate to any bit of this story? For example, the relief, avoidance, or lack of valued direction? Or do you know anyone like George?

What do you notice in terms of the cost to George as he responds to his passengers in these ways? Does it impact his ability to move toward his values?

We would like to suggest an alternative way to respond to passengers that we don't see George using very much. We call this response "openness." An open response is one that eases struggle and allows for the opportunity to continue with values-based actions, while also bringing passengers along for the ride. Let's practice this.

Willingness Exercise (Open)

Aim: To practice a willingness exercise, contrasting the impact of struggle with, absorption with, and willingness regarding painful or difficult thoughts and feelings.

Ensure that everyone has a paper folder or a piece of paper for the exercise. You could also ask participants to write down their "sticky" thoughts on the folder or paper.

Dialogue Example

Sometimes we get so caught up trying to get rid of stuff inside that we end up losing sight of what's important. If we let go of the struggle to get rid of stuff and open ourselves a bit to allow that stuff to be there—not that we have to like it—we can get back to doing what's really important. Now we're going to practice being open to allow thoughts and feelings to be as they are, in this moment.

Pushing Against the Folder Exercise

I invite you to take your folder in both hands. I want you to imagine this folder represents all the difficult thoughts, feelings, memories, and sensations you've been struggling with for so long. And I'd like you to take hold of your folder and grip it as tightly as you can. [Pause.]

Now, I'd like you to hold your folder up in front of your face so you can't see me anymore—bring it up so close to your face that it almost touches your nose. Imagine that this is what it's like to be completely caught up with these thoughts, feelings, or memories.

Now, just notice. What's it like trying to have a conversation or to connect with me while you're all caught up in your thoughts and feelings? Do you feel connected with me, or engaged with me? Are you able to read the expressions on my face? See what I'm doing?

And what's your view of the room like, while you're all caught up in this stuff? [Pause.]

So, while you're completely absorbed in all this stuff, you're missing out on a lot. You're disconnected from the world around you, and you're disconnected from me. Notice, too, that while you're holding on tightly to this stuff, you can't do the things that make your life work. Check it out—grip the folder as tightly as you possibly can.

Can you really connect with loved ones while you're caught up with this stuff? Can you do your job properly?

Now, without letting go of your folder, I want you to try and push it away. Try to get rid of all those difficult thoughts and feelings.

Keep pushing. You can't stand these feelings; you want them to go away; push harder.

Notice how much effort and energy it requires trying to make these thoughts and feelings go away. [Pause.]

So here you are, trying very hard to push away all these painful thoughts and feelings. You've probably tried distracting yourself with TV, music, computers, drink, avoiding people, avoiding work, so forth, and so on.

You've been doing this for years, just pushing and pushing. Are those painful thoughts and feelings going anywhere? [Pause.]

You're able to keep them at arm's length, but what's the cost to you? How does it feel in your shoulders?

While you are doing this, pushing your folder away, would you be able to connect with your friends and family, cook dinner, do your job effectively, or drive your bus of life? Do you think it would be easy to have a conversation and really connect with the other person while you're doing this? [Pause.]

So, trying to push all those feelings away is eating up a lot of effort and energy. This is what you've been doing for so long now, trying to get rid of unpleasant thoughts and feelings. And yet, they keep showing up; they are still having an effect on your life.

Now, rest the folder on your lap for a moment. Just let these thoughts and feelings sit there on your lap. [Pause five seconds.]

How does that feel? Isn't it a lot less effort?

Those painful, distracting thoughts and feelings are still there. But notice the difference: now you can hug someone you love, cook dinner, or drive your bus of life. It's not draining you or tiring you out. [Pause.]

Isn't that easier than constantly trying to push these feelings away or being so caught up with them? [Mime pushing the folder away and holding it up to your nose.]

The difficult feelings are still there. And, of course, you don't want them; who would want all these painful thoughts and feelings? But notice how this stuff is having much less of an impact on you. Now I'm sure in the ideal world you'd like to do this [mime throwing the folder on the floor].

But here's the thing: you've been trying to do that for years. You've clearly put a lot of time, effort, and money into trying to get rid of these thoughts and feelings. And yet, despite all that effort, they're still showing up. They're still here today.

One of the goals of these workshops is to teach you how to be open to experiencing difficult thoughts and feelings instead of fighting with them or trying to avoid them.

After facilitating the exercise, debrief by inviting participant observations about the exercise. Reinforce anything people noticed. Participants may highlight that difficult feelings are still present, in which case the **dialogue example** given below may be useful.

Dialogue Example

How did people find the exercise? What was it like being caught up with those thoughts and feelings? What was it like fighting and pushing away the thoughts and feelings? What did you notice in your body? What couldn't you do while you were pushing the folder away? What was it like placing the folder on your lap, with those difficult thoughts and feelings still there, but not struggling with them? What was it like to drop the struggle?

In these workshops we're learning noticing skills that will enable you to respond to painful thoughts and feelings far more effectively—in such a way that they will have much less impact on and influence over you. We have already covered some techniques, such as focusing on what's important to you and practicing the skill of being mindful and in the present moment, which allows you to think before responding.

Acting Out the Passengers on the Bus Exercise (Open)

Aim: To act out the passengers on the bus metaphor, using the content from the video vignette and running through three key scenarios that represent different responses to passengers. A video demonstration of this exercise is available at http://www.actforpsychosis.com.

Explain to participants that this exercise involves a group role-play of the passengers on the bus metaphor using the content from the video of Paul or George. Emphasize fun aspects of participating, but make it clear that it's okay to just observe. Begin by asking for volunteers:

- **One person needs to act as the driver (either Paul or George).** Have the group decide on the main passengers (for example, worry, paranoia, guilt, and so forth; thoughts like *I'm going crazy* or *I'm a bad father*) based on content from the video vignette.

- **Another three to four people need to act as passengers.** Ask for volunteers to play the role of the driver's passengers. Provide them with sticky notes with the label of their passenger, and remind them of the kinds of things each passenger would say (for example, Paul's "worry" passenger might talk about people recording him or trying to poison his food; George's "guilty" passenger might talk about him being a bad father who passed on his genes).

- **One person needs to act as the valued direction.** Ask the driver to identify the valued direction that the passengers are getting in the way of. Summarize this in one or two words on a large sheet of paper, and ask for a volunteer to hold this representation of the driver's valued direction.

Here are some useful things to keep in mind while doing the role-play:

- Try to ensure clarity around values (defining values rather than goals).

- Tell people how long the exercise will last, and how long they'll be in the roles.

- Try to have at least three passengers, although this number may vary depending on the number of people in the workshop.

- Before starting each scenario, discuss with the driver how the passengers will act out the different responses. For example, ask the driver how he will argue and struggle with the passengers, or how he will act out giving in to the passengers. Give prompts as necessary.

- Due to the emotive nature of the task, it may be useful to have the group come up with ground rules about how to carry out the exercise. For example, make sure the statements from passengers are not too evocative and that the driver feels safe.

- In terms of instructing passengers on what to say, be flexible and allow improvisation. The exercise is often more relevant if they come up with their own comments and actions.

- Link in the different ways that participants reponded during the pushing against the folder exercise.

- Ask the rest of the group to be actively watching as the role-play unfolds.

Fight/Struggle Scenario

In this scenario, have the driver role-play driving the bus (walking around the room with the passengers following) and stopping to fight and struggle (for example, yelling at passengers, arguing with them). Have the passengers behave like passengers (hassling, cajoling, pleading, distracting). Do this for two to four minutes. After the exercise, do the following:

- **Ask for feedback from the bus driver:** How was it to struggle with the passengers? (The facilitator can suggest that no matter how much one argues and fights with passengers, nothing changes the quality of stuckness.)

- **Ask for feedback from the passengers:** Did they feel in control of the driver?

- **Ask for feedback from the values representative:** Did this volunteer feel connected with the bus driver or ignored?
- **Ask for feedback from the wider group:** What did group members notice as observers?

Giving-In Scenario

Ask the driver to again drive the bus, this time role-playing *giving in* to the passengers (for example, agreeing with what they say, trying to make peace with passengers by allowing them to dictate where the bus goes, and so on). Do this for two to four minutes. After the exercise, do the following:

- **Ask for feedback from the bus driver:** How was it to give in to the passengers? What was it like to let go of the steering wheel? Did it feel like the passengers were in control of the bus's direction? Reinforce that it may feel better in the short term, but at the cost of important life areas—that is, being stuck in another way.
- **Ask for feedback from the passengers:** Did they feel in control of the driver?
- **Ask for feedback from the values representative:** Did this person feel connected to the bus driver or ignored?
- **Ask for feedback from the wider group:** What did group members notice as observers?

Openness Scenario

Finally, ask the driver to practice an *openness* response (for example, using skills for noticing the passengers; thanking them for their comments; welcoming them on the bus; allowing them to be on the bus while steering it in a valued direction, with the passengers following behind saying or doing the things they usually say). Do this for two to four minutes. After the exercise, do the following:

- **Ask for feedback from the bus driver:** How was it to focus on values and keep them in mind while the passengers were saying or doing all those things?

- **Ask for feedback from the passengers:** Did they still feel in control of the driver?

- **Ask for feedback from the values representative:** Did this person feel connected to the bus driver or ignored?

- **Ask for feedback from the wider group:** What did group members notice as observers?

Debrief

Ask all participants how they experienced the exercise, and compare and contrast the three different scenarios. Highlight the differences between the first two responses and the openness (willingness) response in terms of key processes: present-moment focus, acceptance, defusion, values clarity, and committed action.

Noticing Exercise (Aware)

Aim: To guide participants through the three-minute breathing space exercise, and to debrief afterward.

Three-Minute Breathing Space Exercise

Now we're going to practice a short breathing exercise that may allow you to step out of automatic mode and reconnect with the present moment.

Find a comfortable, upright position, and either close your eyes or focus on a spot in front of you. Now take a deep breath to bring yourself into the present moment [pause], just noticing whatever you are experiencing right now. Noticing any sensations, be they of discomfort or tension. Noticing your feet on the ground, or, if you're sitting, noticing whatever you are sitting on; notice your clothes against your body and the air against the skin. [Pause five seconds.]

And now, notice whatever is in your mind. Whatever thoughts are here, and as best you can, just observe your thoughts as they are in your mind right now. [Pause.] Now notice whatever you are feeling emotionally. Don't try to change it, but just noticing how you are feeling. [Pause five seconds.]

And now, bring your attention to your breath, just noticing the rise and fall of your stomach as you breathe in [pause], and as you breathe out. [Pause five seconds.]

Notice the cool air flowing in through your nose as you inhale and the warm air as you exhale [pause], as you breathe in and out. [Pause.]

If you find your mind wandering away from your breath, simply bring it back to noticing each breath in, and out, as they follow, one after the other. [Pause five seconds.]

And now, allow your awareness to expand to encompass your breath moving in your body [pause], bringing your awareness to your thinking [pause], and whatever you are feeling emotionally right now. Gently broaden this awareness to notice the whole experience, holding everything in awareness. [Pause five seconds.]

Now bring your attention back to the room; open your eyes if they are closed. Notice what you can see; notice what you can hear. Push your feet into the ground and have a stretch; notice yourself stretching. Welcome back!

After completing the exercise, invite observations from participants. Ask what they noticed and invite curiosity about the experience. Focus on drawing out differences between this experience and automatic-pilot experiences.

Dialogue Example

What did people notice when doing this exercise? Were people able to notice any sensations? Did you notice any thoughts? Were people aware of their mind wandering off during the exercise? Were you able to bring your attention back to noticing your experiences?

Committed Action (Active)

Aim: To set a committed action for the following week.
On the whiteboard write the following:

- Think of one action you could take that would move you toward a value.

- What passengers might get in the way as you try to take this action?

- How might you respond to these passengers?

- Try to practice a noticing exercise during the following week.

Dialogue Example

Think about the important value you identified last week. Can you think of one action you could do next week that would reinforce that this value is important? It doesn't have to be the same action you did last week. You may choose to do something completely different. Keep in mind that this is an opportunity to practice mindful noticing of passengers and your responses to them. If you complete the action, that's icing on the cake.

After reviewing the items on the whiteboard, have the group break into smaller groups, with a facilitator leading each one. Ask participants to complete the committed action worksheet to identify one values-based action they can take the following week that might move them toward their values. Remind people to set a SMART goal.

Within the small groups, facilitators should ask people if they would be willing to tell the others what they plan to do. Also, determine if participants would like one of the facilitators to contact them between sessions for a short five-minute phone call to discuss their committed actions. Make it clear that the phone calls are not designed as a way for the facilitator to check up on whether participants have completed the action, but to serve as reminders of the process, such as mindful noticing and willingness.

Reinforce anything that suggests participants are willing to share their commitments with others. Ask participants to complete the developing aware skills worksheet, and see if they would be willing to practice the three-minute breathing space at least three times during the next week.

Closing the Session

Aim: To bring the group to a close and encourage participants to offer feedback about their experience of the session.

Come back together as a large group and ask for feedback about the workshop session. Ask participants how they generally found the session, and what they found most memorable. Reinforce the importance of attending next week's session.

To prompt feedback, consider writing the following on the whiteboard:

- How did you find the session to be today?

- What did you notice?

- What did you find helpful or unhelpful, or both?
- What was the most memorable thing from today's workshop?

If short on time, you could ask for "popcorn feedback": ask everyone to say one or two words to sum up what they found most memorable from the day's session.

SESSION 3

Acting on Values with Openness, Awareness, and Willingness

The main purpose of session 3 is to link acting on values with noticing and willingness, to practice defusion from experiences, and to get in contact with valued directions. First, facilitators and participants will discuss the purpose of the workshop and what happened in the last session before doing a warm-up exercise. A facilitator will lead the group through the leaves on the stream exercise, followed by an inquiry debrief. The group will then break into small groups to review their committed actions. Then they practice openness using the sticky labels and "having versus buying into thoughts" exercises. The group will then act out the passengers on the bus metaphor with a focus on how one responds to the various passengers. Afterward, a facilitator will lead the group through the three-minute breathing space exercise, after which participants will break into small groups and complete committed action worksheets. The session closes with a discussion of dates for future workshops, and a facilitator encourages participants to attend the next session. The following session outline suggests an order for the topics and time frames. As always, the times given for each segment are approximate.

Timeline

Welcome and introduction	10 minutes
Noticing exercise (aware)	15 minutes
Committed action review	15 minutes
Openness	25 minutes
Acting out the passengers on the bus exercise (open)	25 minutes
Noticing exercise (aware)	10 minutes
Committed action (active)	15 minutes
Closing the session	5 minutes

Materials You'll Need

- Whiteboard
- Paper and pens
- Marker pens
- Folders
- Refreshments
- Committed action worksheets
- Developing Aware Skills Worksheet

Additional Equipment for This Session

- A soft ball
- Sticky notes

Welcome and Introduction

Aim: To welcome participants to session 3 (of 4) of the ACT for recovery workshop.

Remind people that the workshop will run for approximately two hours with a short break halfway through. If required, take care of housekeeping issues (e.g., location of fire escapes, bathrooms). Ask people again to wear name badges. Recap what was covered in session 2 using the whiteboard:

- Thinking about what's important to us (our values)
- How our minds can come up with barriers (passengers)
- Considering the effects of struggling with our minds
- Considering openness as an alternative

Dialogue Example

Here are some of the main topics we've talked about so far in these workshops.

After the review, help participants warm up for the session with a brief exercise. Invite everyone to stand up, and ask them to describe what passengers they noticed during the week and how they responded to them. Facilitators can start by giving their own examples (for example, the "I'm useless," "I can't be bothered," and "anxiety" passengers). Afterward, acknowledge and draw out similarities in the content of people's passengers to set the scene for exercises later in the session.

Dialogue Example

To get us started, we'd like to invite you to do a short warm-up exercise. The person holding the ball briefly describes a passenger he noticed during the week—or another person's passenger, or just a general passenger—and how he responded to it. He then passes the ball to another person, who describes her passenger, and so on, until we've all had a turn.

Noticing Exercise (Aware)

Aim: To introduce and guide people through the exercise, with time to carry out an inquiry afterward.

Dialogue Example

Now we are going to practice a short exercise that will give you an idea of how we can be with and observe our unwanted thoughts, urges, and feelings with openness, without judging them, without holding on to them, and without pushing them away.

You may notice how this process is similar to being with the passengers on the bus: you're practicing noticing when you get caught up with struggling or fixing, and bringing yourself back to having your hands on the steering wheel, deciding where you want to go in your life…even with the passengers there.

Leaves on the Stream Exercise

I invite you to sit in a comfortable yet upright position in your chair, with your feet flat on the floor, your arms and legs uncrossed, and your hands resting in your lap. [Pause.] Let your eyes gently close, or fix them on a point in front of you. [Pause five seconds.] Take a couple of gentle breaths in [pause], and out. [Pause.] Notice the sound and feel of your own breath as you breathe in [pause], and out. [Pause five seconds.]

Now, I'd like you to imagine that you are standing by the bank of a gently flowing stream watching the water flow. [Pause.] Imagine feeling the ground beneath you, the sounds of the water flowing past, and the way the stream looks as you watch it. [Pause five seconds.] Imagine that there are leaves from trees, of all different shapes, sizes, and colors, floating past on the stream. And you are just watching these float on the stream. This is all you need to do for the time being. [Pause five seconds.]

Start to become aware of your thoughts, feelings, or sensations. [Pause.] Each time you notice a thought, feeling, or sensation, imagine placing it on a leaf and letting it float down the stream. [Pause five seconds.] Do this regardless of whether the thoughts, feelings, or sensations are positive or negative, pleasurable or painful. [Pause.] Even if they are the most wonderful thoughts, place them on a leaf and let them float by. [Pause five seconds.]

If your thoughts stop, just watch the stream. Sooner or later your thoughts should start up again. [Pause five seconds.] Allow the stream to flow at its own rate. [Pause.] Notice any urges to speed up or slow down the stream, and let these be on leaves as well. Let the stream flow how it will. [Pause five seconds.]

If you have thoughts, feelings, or sensations about doing this exercise, place these on leaves as well. [Pause five seconds.]

If a leaf gets stuck or won't go away, let it hang around. For a little while, all you are doing is observing this experience; there is no need to force the leaf down the stream. [Pause five seconds.]

If you find yourself getting caught up with a thought or feeling, such as boredom or impatience, simply acknowledge it. Say to yourself, "Here's a feeling of boredom," or "Here's a feeling of impatience." Then place those words on a leaf, and let them float on by. [Pause five seconds.]

You are just observing each experience and placing it on a leaf on the stream. It is normal and natural to lose track of this exercise, and it will keep happening. When you notice yourself losing track, just bring yourself back to watching the leaves on the stream. [Pause ten seconds.]

Notice the stream, and place any thoughts, feelings, or sensations on the leaves and let them gently float down the stream. [Pause five seconds.]

Finally, allow the image of the stream to dissolve, and slowly bring your attention back into sitting in the chair, in this room. [Pause.] Gently open your eyes and notice what you can see. Notice what you can hear. Push your feet onto the floor and have a stretch. Notice yourself stretching. Welcome back.

After completing the exercise, invite observations from participants. Explore what people noticed in terms of their tendency to get hooked by thoughts and feelings and their ability to bring themselves back to observing leaves.

Reinforce noticing, and draw their attention to how easily our minds can get hooked; stress that observing experiences is a choice, and that it takes active noticing.

Some people may report that they wanted to hold on to positive thoughts rather than place them on leaves. While validating this response, highlight that the aim is to observe the natural flow of thoughts, whether positive or negative, allowing them to come and go.

Dialogue Example

What did people notice while doing this exercise? What types of experiences hooked you? What was it like to let go of experiences so they could come and go without you holding on to them?

Committed Action Review

Aim: To review the committed action worksheets that participants completed at the end of the previous session and to explore whether people had the opportunity to increase openness responses.

On the whiteboard write the following:

- Think of the value you identified and the action linked to this value.

- Did you notice any passengers show up in relation to this action?

- What was your experience of the mindfulness practice?

Then break into small groups with one facilitator to lead each group. Encourage participants to describe what passengers they encountered and what they noticed about the committed-action process. Reinforce all efforts to take committed actions in valued directions, as well as any noticing on the part of participants. Reinforce all steps taken in or inclinations for valued directions, as these are part of building repertoires of effective behavior.

With those participants who had difficulty engaging in committed actions, reinforce any feedback they give in relation to thinking about taking action, such as small plans, inclinations, and so forth. Similarly, reinforce any noticing of barriers to doing the task, of struggling, and so on. This is a good opportunity to mention using defusion/acceptance and mindfulness skills when facing barriers, as well as the concept of openness to having unwanted experiences that are part of taking committed actions in valued directions.

Dialogue Example

We would like to hear how things have gone with increasing your openness since the last session. What committed actions did you take? And what was that like? What passengers did you notice? How did you respond to them? What did you do that let the passengers be while you moved in your valued direction?

[Invite observations from participants.] How did the mindfulness practice go? Were you able to fit the practice into your usual routines? What did people notice?

Openness

Aim: To provide participants experience with practicing defusion and openness toward difficult experiences.

Explain the sticky labels exercise to participants. Facilitators can lead by example by writing one of their sticky thoughts on a label and wearing it. Once everyone has written on their labels and stuck them to their chest, invite participants to walk around the room and look at each other's labels without commenting on them.

After the exercise take a break, and then debrief to get people's experiences, to draw out commonalities of experience, and to link the idea of openness with passengers. Try to do this exercise before the break so participants can wear the labels during the break.

Sticky Labels Exercise

We're going to do an exercise now that involves coming into contact with some of the sticky, tricky things our minds come up with. The kinds of things that really grab our attention in a way that stops us from doing the things that matter to us.

I'd like you to spend a few moments thinking about the kinds of things that you notice your passengers saying about you that really grab your attention. These are often the critical, judgmental, negative things we say about ourselves.

If you're anything like me, you'll probably notice an urge to hide these things and not let anyone know about them: "It's too shameful!" or "What if it's true?" or "I couldn't bear other people knowing!" These are often the kinds of things our passengers will convince us of, and it's their way of keeping what they say hidden away.

Today we're going to do something a bit different than what we might normally do when we're on automatic pilot. I'm going to ask you to think about one of the things that your passengers often say to you that you'd feel comfortable sharing with other people in the group. It doesn't have to be a huge disclosure, but perhaps something that takes you slightly out of your comfort zone.

Then, see if you can reduce it to one or two words. Let me give you an example. A passenger of mine often says, "You don't think about other people enough—you're selfish!"

So, on my label I'm going to write "selfish."

[Ask participants to write their sticky thought on the label and put it on their clothes. Encourage them to write down a maximum of two words.]

Now, as you do this task, I'd like you to watch out for and notice any passengers that show up. Notice any urges to either go along with what the passengers are saying or to fight or struggle with them. See if you can make some room and space for them, and mindfully engage in the task at hand.

Once we have all written our labels, then we're going to ask everyone to stand up and walk around the room. Take this opportunity to look at the person, read their labels, and notice what comes to mind. Try not to explain why you've written what you have on your label, and try not to comment or "rescue" other people when you see what is written on their labels.

We're going to wear these labels while we take a break.

After the break, invite observations about the exercise:

- What did you notice?
- Did anyone notice passengers getting vocal?
- What feelings, emotions, and sensations showed up?
- What was it like noticing what other people's passengers say?

Having vs. Buying Into Thoughts Exercise

This exercise helps participants practice defusion techniques. On the whiteboard write the following:

- I can't be bothered.
- It's all going to go wrong.
- I'm going to look stupid.
- I'm no good at this.

You can choose the above statements, or, if more appropriate, you could use one of the examples of sticky thoughts discussed in the sticky labels exercise.

Ask participants to read the statements written on the whiteboard in their head, using the tone that normally goes along with such thoughts (heavy, grim, shrill, and so forth), and notice how it makes them feel. Then, ask them to put "I'm having the thought that…" in front of each sentence, or have facilitators write the phrase before each statement on the whiteboard, and then ask participants to reread the statements in their heads. Ask them whether they noticed any difference between the first time and second time reading the statements. Finally, ask them to add "I notice I'm having the thought that…" to each phrase and to reread them. Ask them again to notice any differences.

Dialogue Example

Sometimes our passengers—our thoughts, feelings, and sensations—seem so real and powerful. We may not be able to get rid of these passengers, but we can notice other aspects of them and change our relationship with them.

After completing the exercise, invite observations from participants. Ask what they noticed and invite curiosity about the experience. Focus on drawing out differences between how participants responded to the three different statements. Point out that by the third iteration, often the original thought loses its impact and power, and there is more space to choose how to respond. Link this exercise to the passengers on the bus metaphor by asking, "Do you think it would be helpful to have this kind of space from your passengers?"

Acting Out the Passengers on the Bus Metaphor (Open)

Aim: To act out the passengers on the bus metaphor, ideally using content from a participant's example; otherwise you can make up an example or use Paul's or George's example from the previous session. A video demonstration of the passengers on the bus exercise is available at http://www.actforpsychosis.com.

Explain to participants that you are going to be role-playing the passengers on the bus metaphor again, but this time you will ideally be using content from a participant's example. Participants will have the opportunity to be the driver and to try out three different responses to the passengers. Emphasize fun aspects of participating, but make it clear that it's okay to just observe the exercise.

Dialogue Example

Does anyone have an example they'd like to act out, maybe something over the last week that we've just been talking about?

[If nobody is forthcoming, the facilitator could ask:] Does anyone have an example they would be willing to direct someone else to act out?

If no one offers an example, act out a general example with common passengers—ones that participants reported in previous sessions. Or, use the example of being in and contributing to a group—a common experience for all participants!

Then ask for volunteers:

- **One person needs to act as the driver (either Paul or George).** Have the group decide on the main passengers (for example, worry, paranoia, guilt, and so forth; thoughts like *I'm going crazy* or *I'm a bad father*) based on content from the video vignette.

- **Another three to four people need to act as passengers.** Ask for volunteers to play the role of the driver's passengers. Provide them with sticky notes with the label of their passenger, and remind them of the kinds of things each passenger would say (for example, Paul's "worry" passenger might talk about people recording him or trying to poison his food; George's "guilty" passenger might talk about him being a bad father who passed on his genes).

- **One person needs to act as the valued direction.** Ask the driver to identify the valued direction that the passengers are getting in the way of. Summarize this in one or two words on a large sheet of paper, and ask for a volunteer to hold this representation of the driver's valued direction.

Here are some useful things to keep in mind while doing the role-play:

- Try to ensure clarity around values (defining values rather than goals).

- Tell people how long the exercise will last, and how long they'll be in the roles.

- Be aware that the number of people in the room may affect the number of passengers on the bus.

- Due to the emotive nature of the task, it may be useful to have the group come up with ground rules about how to carry out the exercise. For example, make sure the statements from passengers are not too evocative and that the driver feels safe.

- In terms of instructing passengers on what to say, be flexible and allow improvisation. The exercise is often more relevant if they come up with their own comments and actions.

Fight/Struggle Scenario

In this scenario, have the driver role-play driving the bus (walking around the room with the passengers following) and stopping to fight and struggle (for example, yelling at passengers, arguing with them). Have the passengers behave like passengers (hassling, cajoling, pleading, distracting). Do this for two to four minutes. After the exercise, do the following:

- **Ask for feedback from the bus driver:** How was it to struggle with the passengers? (The facilitator can suggest that no matter how much one argues and fights with passengers, nothing changes the quality of stuckness.)

- **Ask for feedback from the passengers:** Did they feel in control of the driver?

- **Ask for feedback from the values representative:** Did this volunteer feel connected with the bus driver or ignored?

- **Ask for feedback from the wider group:** What did group members notice as observers?

Giving-In Scenario

Ask the driver to again drive the bus, this time role-playing *giving in* to the passengers (for example, agreeing with what they say, trying to make peace with passengers by allowing them to dictate where the bus goes, and so on). Do this for two to four minutes. After the exercise, do the following:

- **Ask for feedback from the bus driver:** How was it to give in to the passengers? What was it like to let go of the steering wheel? Did it feel like the passengers were in control of the bus's direction? Reinforce the qualities that it may feel better in the short term, but at the cost of important life areas—that is, being stuck in another way.

- **Ask for feedback from the passengers:** Did they feel in control of the driver?

- **Ask for feedback from the values representative:** Did this person feel connected to the bus driver or ignored?

- **Ask for feedback from the wider group:** What did group members notice as observers?

Openness Scenario

Finally, ask the driver to practice an *openness* response (for example, using skills for noticing the passengers; thanking them for their comments; welcoming them on the bus; allowing them to be on the bus while steering it in a valued direction, with the passengers following behind saying or doing the things they usually say). Do this for two to four minutes. After the exercise, do the following:

- **Ask for feedback from the bus driver:** How was it to focus on values and keep them in mind while the passengers were saying or doing all those things?

- **Ask for feedback from the passengers:** Did they still feel in control of the driver?

- **Ask for feedback from the values representative:** Did this person feel connected to the bus driver or ignored?

- **Ask for feedback from the wider group:** What did group members notice as observers?

Debrief

Ask all participants how they experienced the exercise, and compare and contrast the three different scenarios. Highlight the differences between the first two responses and the openness (willingness) response in terms of key processes: present-moment focus, acceptance, defusion, values clarity, and committed action.

Noticing Exercise (Aware)

Aim: To guide participants through the three-minute breathing space exercise, and to debrief afterward.

Three-Minute Breathing Space Exercise

Now we're going to practice a short breathing exercise that may allow you to step out of automatic mode and reconnect with the present moment.

Find a comfortable, upright position, and either close your eyes or focus on a spot in front of you. Now take a deep breath to bring yourself into the present moment [pause], just noticing whatever you are experiencing right now. Noticing any sensations, be they of discomfort or tension. Noticing your feet on the ground, or, if you're sitting, noticing whatever you are sitting on; notice your clothes against your body and the air against the skin. [Pause five seconds.]

And now, notice whatever is in your mind. Whatever thoughts are here, and as best you can, just observe your thoughts as they are in your mind right now. [Pause.] Now notice whatever you are feeling emotionally. Don't try to change it, but just notice how you are feeling. [Pause five seconds.]

And now, bring your attention to your breath, just noticing the rise and fall of your stomach as you breathe in [pause], and as you breathe out. [Pause five seconds.] Notice the cool air flowing in through your nose as you inhale and the warm air as you exhale [pause], as you breathe in and out. [Pause.]

If you find your mind wandering away from your breath, simply bring it back to noticing each breath in, and out, as they follow, one after the other. [Pause five seconds.]

And now, allow your awareness to expand to encompass your breath moving in your body [pause], bringing your awareness to your thinking [pause], and whatever you are feeling emotionally right now. Gently broaden this awareness to notice the whole experience, holding everything in awareness. [Pause five seconds.]

Now bring your attention back to the room; open your eyes if they are closed. Notice what you can see; notice what you can hear. Push your feet into the ground and have a stretch; notice yourself stretching. Welcome back!

After completing the exercise, invite observations from participants. Ask what they noticed and invite curiosity about the experience. Focus on drawing out differences between this experience and automatic-pilot experiences.

Dialogue Example

What did people notice when doing this exercise? Were people able to notice any sensations? Did you notice any thoughts? Were people aware of their mind wandering off during the exercise? Were you able to bring your attention back to noticing your experiences?

Committed Action (Active)

Aim: To set a committed action for the following week.

On the whiteboard write the following:

- Think of one action you could take that would move you toward a value.

- What passengers might get in the way as you try to take this action?

- How might you respond to these passengers?

- Try to practice a noticing exercise during the following week.

Dialogue Example

Think about the important value you identified in session 1. Can you think of one action you could do during the next week that would reinforce that this value is important? It doesn't have to be the same action you took last week. You may choose to do something completely different. Keep in mind that this is an opportunity to practice mindful noticing of passengers and your response to them, and to practice being with passengers as part of an openness response.

After reviewing the items on the whiteboard, have the group break into smaller groups, with a facilitator leading each one. Ask participants to complete the committed action worksheet to identify one values-based action they can take the following week that might move them toward their values. Remind people to set a SMART goal.

Within the small groups, facilitators should ask people if they would be willing to tell the others what they plan to do. Also, determine if participants would like one of the facilitators to contact them between sessions for a short five-minute phone call to discuss their committed actions. Make it clear that the phone calls are not designed as a way for the facilitator to check up on whether they have completed the action, but to serve as reminders of the process, such as mindful noticing and willingness.

Reinforce anything that suggests participants are willing to share their commitments with others. Ask participants to complete the developing aware skills worksheet, and see if they would be willing to practice the leaves on the stream exercise at least three times during the next week.

Closing the Session

Aim: To bring the group to a close and encourage participants to offer feedback about their experience of the session.

Come back together as a large group and ask for feedback about the workshop session. Ask participants how they generally found the session, and what they found most memorable. Reinforce the importance of attending next week's session.

To prompt feedback, consider writing the following on the whiteboard:

- How did you find the session to be today?

- What did you notice?

- What did you find helpful or unhelpful, or both?

- What was the most memorable thing from today's workshop?

If short on time, you could ask for "popcorn feedback": ask everyone to say one or two words to sum up what they found most memorable from the day's session.

SESSION 4

Bringing It All Together—Open, Aware, and Active

The main purpose of session 4 (of 4) is to review progress so far and support the concepts of open, aware, and active; to review the content of the group; to provide an opportunity to practice exercises; and to reinforce group participation. First, facilitators and participants will discuss what has been covered in the workshop before doing a warm-up exercise. A facilitator will lead the group through the mindful walking exercise, followed by an inquiry debrief. The group will then break into small groups to review committed actions. Then they will practice noticing others' values. The group will then participate in the key messages exercise, which works with open, aware, and active, and recap the passengers on the bus metaphor, with an emphasis on how participants can "be" with their passengers. Then the session moves on to a review of what participants have learned thus far and where to go from here, followed by completing the driving license worksheet. A facilitator will lead the group through the "clouds in the sky" exercise with an inquiry debrief. Finally, the group will discuss how to tie together everything they've learned. The session closes with a discussion of dates for the booster workshop sessions, and a facilitator will encourage participants to attend these. The following session outline suggests an order for the topics and time frames. As always, the times given for each segment are approximate.

Timeline

Welcome and introduction	10 minutes
Noticing exercise (aware)	15 minutes
Committed action review	15 minutes
Values (active)	10 minutes
Key messages exercise	20 minutes
Passengers on the bus review	15 minutes
Review and moving forward	15 minutes
Noticing exercise (aware)	10 minutes
Tying it all together	5 minutes
Closing the session	5 minutes

Materials You'll Need

- Laptop and projector
- Paper and pens
- Marker pens
- Folders
- Refreshments
- Driving license worksheets
- Developing Aware Skills Worksheet

Additional Equipment for This Session

- A soft ball
- Laminated cards or sticky notes for key messages exercise
- Three pieces of flip-chart paper with the headings "open," "aware," and "active"

- Sticky dots or stars and adhesive putty
- Certificates

Welcome and Introduction

Aim: To welcome participants to session 4 (of 4) of the ACT for recovery workshop.

Remind participants of what has been covered in the workshop so far by working through the key points on the whiteboard:

- Thinking about what's important to us (our values)
- How our minds can come up with barriers (passengers)
- Considering the effects of struggling with our minds
- Considering openness as an alternative
- Noticing our passengers but not acting on them

Dialogue Example

Here are some of the main topics we have talked about so far in these workshops.

After the review, help participants warm up for the session with a brief exercise. Invite everyone to stand up, and ask them to describe what values they have worked toward in the workshop sessions. Facilitators can give examples of their own values and what they have worked on.

Dialogue Example

To get us started, we'd like to invite you to do a short warm-up exercise. The person holding the ball says what values she has worked toward in the workshop and then passes the ball to another person, who describes his values, and so on, until we've all had a turn.

Noticing Exercise (Aware)

Aim: To introduce and guide people through the mindful walking exercise, leaving enough time to carry out an inquiry afterward.

When doing the mindful walking exercise, it's helpful to have all participants walk in the same direction, either clockwise or counterclockwise. Ask people to keep their eyes open during the exercise. You may also advise people wearing high heels that it might be helpful to take their shoes off, if they are willing.

Dialogue Example

In this next exercise we're going to use the movement of our own bodies to explore our awareness. I invite you to notice the changing sensations in your body and to open your awareness to what your body is telling you.

When doing this exercise, try to adopt a sense of curiosity about your own experiences. We do this exercise to explore our shifting attention, bringing our attention to the simple task of walking. All of us walk every day, often on automatic pilot, not noticing what we are doing or where we are going. We will do this exercise without a goal or the aim of getting anywhere, rather we will simply notice the sensations in our body, the activity of our mind, and the regularity of our breath.

Mindful Walking Exercise

Start by standing with your feet flat on the ground, and bring your attention to the soles of your feet. [Pause.] Wiggle your toes if this helps to focus your awareness. [Pause.] Start to become aware of your weight passing through the soles of your feet into the ground. Notice all the delicate movements that happen in order to keep us balanced and upright. [Pause.]

Now, start walking at a slow pace. Try not to change the way you walk; simply be aware of the way you are walking. [Pause.] Your body may do a funny wobble as soon as you become aware of yourself. Don't worry, that's a natural effect. [Pause five seconds.]

Direct your attention to the soles of your feet, being aware of the constant patterns of landing and lifting. [Pause five seconds.] Be aware of your foot as the heel first contacts the ground. Notice how your foot rolls forward onto the ball, and then lifts and travels through the air again. [Pause.] Visualize your feet going through this pattern as you walk. [Pause five seconds.]

Try to be aware of all the different sensations in your feet [pause], not just the contact with the soles of your feet but the connection between the toes [pause], and the sensation of your feet against the fabric of your socks or shoes. [Pause.] Try to let your feet be as relaxed as possible. [Pause five seconds.]

Now, direct your attention to your ankles. [Pause.] Notice the sensation in your joints. Allow your ankles to be relaxed. Try not to resist the movement of your ankles in any way. Now, become aware of your lower legs [pause], your shins [pause], and your calves as you walk. [Pause five seconds.]

You might notice that your mind wanders while doing this exercise. This is common, and it may happen again and again. If it does, try to bring your attention back to the exercise of walking and focusing on your body. [Pause five seconds.]

Now, expand your awareness to your thighs [pause]; notice how your clothing feels on your skin. [Pause.] Be aware of the front and rear thigh muscles. [Pause.] Become aware of the whole of your pelvis [pause], and notice all the movements that are going on in your pelvis as you walk. Notice how one hip moves forward, and then the other [pause]; one hip lifts, the other sinks, and you walk. [Pause.] Just keep walking and noticing your body as you do this exercise. [Pause five seconds.]

Next, notice your shoulders. [Pause.] Try to see how they are moving in rhythm as you walk. [Pause.] Are they moving opposite to your hips? Are your arms simply hanging by your sides and swinging naturally? [Pause five seconds.]

Lastly, come to a natural stop and just experience yourself standing. [Pause.] Notice what it's like to no longer be mobile. [Pause five seconds.] Notice once more the balancing act that's going on to keep you upright. [Pause.] Feeling once again the weight traveling down through the soles of your feet into the ground. Congratulate yourself for your intention to practice mindful walking, no matter how many times your mind was pulled away from the walk, or how "well" you thought your practice went today. Just notice that the intention to be mindful is the key to practice. Welcome back.

After completing the exercise, invite observations from participants. Explore what people noticed in terms of their tendency to get hooked by thoughts and feelings and their ability to bring themselves back to observing mindful walking.

Reinforce noticing, and draw participants' attention to how easily our minds can get hooked; stress that observing experiences is a choice, and that it takes active noticing.

Dialogue Example

What did people notice when doing this exercise? What was it like paying attention to walking like this? What did you notice while walking really slowly? Did people notice where their mind went during this exercise?

Committed Action Review (Active)

Aim: To review the committed action worksheets that participants completed at the end of the previous session and to explore whether people had the opportunity to increase openness responses.

On the whiteboard write the following:

- Think of the value you identified and the action linked to this value.
- Did you notice any passengers show up in relation to this action?
- What was your experience of the mindfulness practice?

Then break into small groups, with one facilitator to lead each group. Encourage participants to describe what passengers they encountered and what they noticed about the committed-action process. Reinforce all efforts to take committed actions in valued directions, as well as any noticing on the part of participants. Reinforce all steps taken in or inclinations for valued directions, as these are part of building repertoires of effective behavior.

With those participants who had difficulty engaging in committed actions, reinforce any feedback they give in relation to thinking about taking action, such as small plans, inclinations, and so forth. Similarly, reinforce any noticing of barriers to doing the task, of struggling, and so on. This is then a good opportunity to mention using defusion/acceptance and mindfulness skills when facing barriers, as well as the concept of openness to having unwanted experiences that are part of taking committed actions in valued directions.

Dialogue Example

We would like to hear how things have gone with increasing your openness since the last session. What committed actions did you take? And what was that like? What passengers did you notice? How did you respond to them? What did you do that let the passengers be while you moved in your valued direction?

[Invite observations from participants.] How did the mindfulness practice go? Were you able to fit the practice into your usual routines? What did people notice?

Reinforce noticing, and draw participants' attention to how easily our mind can get hooked; stress that observing experiences is a choice, and that it takes active noticing.

Noticing Exercise (Aware)

Aim: To encourage participants to describe what they have noticed their fellow members doing over the course of the workshop sessions that reflects what is important to them (their values).

Dialogue Example

Now we're going to get in touch with our values again by having others notice and acknowledge them.

Ask participants to pair up and write down one or two things (for example, behaviors) they have noticed in the other person over the course of workshop sessions that they think reflects what is important (values) to this person. Ask that they don't discuss these with their partner. It may be helpful to remind the group that values are statements about what we want to be doing with our lives, what we want to stand for, and how we want to behave on an ongoing basis.

Facilitators may have to prompt participants or remind them about discussions in previous sessions (for example, "Bob volunteering to act out his passengers indicates that participating is important to him," or "I noticed that Joy has made more effort to reduce her drinking; to me this links with her values." Ask participants to think about what values drive these behaviors. Come together as one group again, and ask participants to offer one behavior they noticed their partner exhibit over the past four weeks and what value they think it reflects.

Afterward, invite participants to reflect on the exercise:

- What was it like to have someone notice your actions and values?

- Did what was said reflect what is important to you?

- Was the action or behavior in line with your values, or did it identify a value that you previously had not thought about?

Key Messages Exercise

Aim: To remind participants of all the exercises covered in the workshop sessions so far and to sort them into the three categories of open, aware, and active.

For the key messages exercise, it can be helpful to either write the different exercises on sticky notes or print and laminate them if you are going to use them often (see the list of exercises below and appendix 13 for copies of key messages cards).

Open

- Passengers on the bus exercise
- Committed actions (homework)
- Pushing against the folder exercise
- Having vs. buying into thoughts exercise
- Sticky labels exercise

Aware

- Mindfulness of breath and body exercise
- Mindful stretch exercise
- Mindful eating exercise
- Three-minute breathing space exercise
- Leaves on the stream exercise
- Mindful walking exercise
- Clouds in the sky exercise
- Videos of Paul and George
- Weekly telephone call from facilitator
- Having vs. buying into thoughts exercise
- Noticing others' values exercise

Active

- Coming to the workshops
- Choosing valued directions
- SMART goals
- Committed action (homework)
- Having vs. buying into thoughts exercise
- Passengers on the bus exercise

Write the three following headings at the top of three pieces of flip-chart paper:

1. **Open:** Willingness, making space/being with
2. **Aware:** Mindful awareness/present-moment focus
3. **Active:** Taking steps toward values/doing what matters

Spread the laminated cards or sticky notes across a table. Ask participants to take the key messages and place them under one of the three headings they feel that particular exercise falls under. Remind them that some of the exercises may fit in more than one category, so the same exercise may show up under multiple headings.

Facilitators then walk around the room with participants to review each of the three categories, discuss people's choices, and clarify the correct placement of the exercises. If an exercise has been placed incorrectly under one heading, the facilitator can ask the group whether they are sure of the fit and encourage a discussion about the correct placement.

Next, using stickers, ask participants to vote on the exercise that stood out for them the most or that they found most useful. Review with the whole group which exercises were the most popular and the possible reasons why (for example, "What was it that made this exercise stand out?").

Sometimes people forget or don't know what a particular exercise is called, so it can be helpful to first go through all the cards and sticky notes with the whole group to check understanding and clarify as necessary. We also suggest allocating five to six stickers per person for voting on the most useful exercises.

Passengers on the Bus Review

Aim: To recap the passengers on the bus metaphor.

Ask participants to highlight the key elements of the metaphor, providing prompts if necessary.

Dialogue Example

Throughout the workshop sessions we have referred to the passengers on the bus metaphor. If you were to describe this metaphor to a friend or loved one, what would you say? What parts of the metaphor were most relevant to you?

During this review, the facilitator should encourage participants to think about and identify ways of being with their passengers. Ask participants to highlight the ways they have learned to deal with passengers as a result of attending the workshops. Write the suggestions below on the whiteboard, as well as any others participants suggest:

- Be clear about the direction you want your bus to go.
- Notice that you have a choice about where you steer the bus.
- Understand that passengers are just passengers.
- Being mindful can help us notice the choices available to us.
- Fighting and struggling with passengers can take you away from what's really important.
- An alternative can be making space for passengers and allowing them to come along for the ride.

Dialogue Example

Did anyone do anything different over the last few weeks that they hadn't done previously? Did anyone notice things they would like to do differently? If you had the choice, what can you see yourself doing differently over the next six months?

It can be helpful to type up and print out cards of all the suggestions from each workshop on how to be with passengers; people can take these and carry them around with them.

Review and Moving Forward

Aim: To allow the participants an opportunity to reflect on what they learned in the workshop sessions.

Ask participants to give examples of what they can take away from the workshop using these prompts:

- What have you noticed?
- How have you responded?
- What was it like for you when you first came to the workshop?
- What's it like now?
- How can you take things forward?

Driving License Worksheet

The driving license worksheet encourages participants to think about how they can put into practice what they learned from the workshop, and make committed actions.

Dialogue Example

Over the past four weeks we have asked you to identify actions that are linked to your values. We would like you to continue these committed actions over the next few months. You can plan these actions on the form that we call your "driving license."

Try to identify long-term goals that you would like to work toward. You can choose a valued goal you already identified or a different one you would like to move toward. Write this valued goal in the "my life goals are" section. Try to identify SMART goals that will take you in this valued direction. Then identify the values linked to these actions and life goals. Then, flip over the sheet and identify the passengers that may get in the way of you moving toward these values.

After explaining the process of filling out the worksheet, break into small groups. One facilitator goes with each group and helps each participant fill out the worksheet. Participants write their life goals, actions, and values on side one of the worksheet and passengers on side two. Then come back together as one group. Ask for feedback about the process of completing the worksheet (for example, "What was easy?" and "What was hard?").

Noticing Exercise (Aware)

Aim: To introduce and guide participants through the clouds in the sky exercise, leaving enough time for an inquiry afterward.

Dialogue Example

Before we finish, we'd like to invite you to do one final noticing exercise. It is similar to the leaves on the stream exercise we did last week. It gives you an idea of how we can be with and observe our unwanted thoughts and feelings, rather than struggling with them.

Clouds in the Sky Exercise

First, get in a comfortable position in your chair. Sit upright with your feet flat on the floor, your arms and legs uncrossed, and your hands resting on your lap. [Pause.] Allow your eyes to close, or fix them on a point in front of you. [Pause five seconds.] Take a couple of gentle breaths in and out. [Pause.] Notice the sensation of your own breath as you breathe in and out. [Pause five seconds.]

Now, try to imagine you are lying on a grassy hill on a warm spring day. [Pause.] Imagine feeling the ground beneath you [pause], the smell of the grass [pause], and the sounds of nearby trees blowing in the wind. [Pause five seconds.] Now, imagine you are looking up at the sky, watching clouds pass by. [Pause.] Start to become conscious of your thoughts and feelings. [Pause.] Each time a thought pops into your head, imagine placing it on one of these clouds and allowing it to float on by. [Pause.] If you think in words or images, place these on a cloud, and let them float by. [Pause five seconds.]

The goal is to continue watching the sky and to allow the clouds to keep moving by. [Pause.] Try not to change what shows up on the clouds in any way. If the clouds disappear or you go somewhere else mentally, just stop and notice this happening, and gently bring yourself back to watching the clouds in the sky. [Pause.]

If you have any thoughts or feelings about doing this exercise, place these on clouds as well. [Pause.] If your thoughts stop, just watch the sky and the clouds. Sooner or later your thoughts should start up again. [Pause five seconds.]

You are just observing each thought or feeling as a word or an image on a cloud. [Pause.] It is normal and natural to lose track of this exercise, and it will keep happening. When you notice yourself losing track, just bring yourself back to watching the clouds in the sky. [Pause.]

Let the clouds float at their own pace, and place any thought, feeling, sensation, or image that comes to mind on a cloud and allow it to float on by. [Pause five seconds.] When a thought hooks you, place that on a cloud and let it float by. [Pause.]

Finally, bring your attention back to your breathing. [Pause five seconds.] Notice again the steady rhythm of your breath that is with you all the time. [Pause five seconds.] Then, bring your awareness back to sitting in the chair, in this room. [Pause.] Gently open your eyes and notice what you can see. Push your feet onto the floor and have a stretch; notice yourself stretching. Welcome back.

After completing the exercise, invite observations from participants. Explore what people noticed in terms of their tendency to get hooked by thoughts and feelings and bringing themselves back to observing the clouds.

Reinforce noticing and draw participants' attention to how easily our minds can get hooked; stress that observing our experiences is a choice, and that it takes active noticing.

Some people may report that they wanted to hold on to positive thoughts rather than place them on clouds, but this can defeat the purpose of the exercise; the aim is to observe the natural flow of thoughts, whether positive or negative, allowing them to come and go.

Dialogue Example

What did people notice while doing this exercise? What types of experiences hooked you? What was it like to let go of experiences so they could come and go without you holding on to them?

Tying It All Together

Aim: To summarize the key messages of the workshop.

Dialogue Example

There may be times both here in the workshop and at home when you experience thoughts and feelings that try to convince you that it's all too much and too difficult, and you don't feel like trying anymore.

Even if you start to think about giving up on a valued direction, try to continue moving toward it. You can be the driver of your bus and take all the passengers with you. You have already experienced in these workshop sessions that thoughts and feelings come and go, but the progress you make toward your goals will be ongoing. This is what really matters.

Ultimately you are in control of the direction of your life, like a bus driver, even if you can't control what kind of feelings, thoughts, or worries come along with you. Act on your values rather than your fears. Do what you care about, in spite of the thoughts and feelings that show up. That is what you truly can control.

Closing the Session

Aim: To gather feedback from the group and reinforce the idea of attending future booster sessions.

Come back together as a large group and ask for feedback about the last four weeks. Ask participants how they generally found the workshop to be and what they found most memorable. Reinforce the importance of attending booster sessions, and remind people of the dates.

To prompt feedback, consider writing the following on the whiteboard:

- How did you find the session to be today?

- What did you notice?

- What did you find helpful or unhelpful, or both?

- What was the most memorable thing from today's session and the last four weeks?

After receiving feedback, hand out certificates to celebrate that group members have completed the workshops. We also find it is helpful to provide printouts with the booster session dates.

Booster Session 1

The main purpose of booster session 1 is to review progress since the end of the last workshop; to support open, aware, and active skills; to review the content of the workshops; and to provide an opportunity to practice exercises. First, facilitators and participants will discuss what the workshops are about before doing a warm-up exercise. A facilitator will lead the group through the mindfulness of breath and body exercise, followed by an inquiry debrief. The group will then review the passengers on the bus metaphor before breaking into small groups to review committed actions. After gathering together again as a large group, facilitators will recap values by using values cards. Following this, facilitators and participants will review open, aware, and active skills. The group will once again break into small groups to fill out committed action worksheets. The session closes with a discussion of dates for the final booster session, and a facilitator encourages participants to attend this booster session. The following session outline suggests an order for the topics and time frames. As always, the times given for each segment are approximate.

Timeline

Welcome and introduction	10 minutes
Noticing exercise (aware)	15 minutes
Passengers on the bus review	5 minutes
Committed action review	10 minutes
Values exercise	15 minutes
Skills refresher	40–50 minutes
Committed action (active)	10 minutes
Closing the session	5 minutes

Materials You'll Need

- Whiteboard
- Paper and pens
- Marker pens
- Refreshments
- Committed action worksheets
- Developing Aware Skills Worksheet

Additional Equipment for This Session

- A soft ball
- Values cards for values exercise (these can be downloaded for free at http://www.louisehayes.com.au/free-resources-for-professionals)

Welcome and Introduction

Aim: To welcome participants to booster session 1 (of 2) of the ACT for recovery workshop.

Remind people that the workshop will run for approximately two hours with a short break halfway through. If required, take care of housekeeping issues (e.g., location of fire escapes, bathrooms). Ask people again to wear name badges. Remind people of the purpose of the workshop by listing the following points on the whiteboard and reading through them:

- Developing life direction
- Increasing awareness of obstacles
- Learning the skills of open, aware, and active
- Connecting with each other and having fun

Dialogue Example

Just as a reminder, here are some of the key points we've covered over the course of these workshops.

After the review, help participants warm up for the session with a brief exercise. Invite everyone to stand up, and ask them to describe what passengers they noticed during the week and how they responded to them. Facilitators can start by giving their own examples (for example, the "I'm useless," "I can't be bothered," and "anxiety" passengers). Afterward, acknowledge and draw out similarities in the content of people's passengers to set the scene for exercises later in the session.

Dialogue Example

To get us started, we'd like to invite you to do a short warm-up exercise. The person holding the ball briefly describes a passenger she noticed during the week—or another person's passenger, or just a general passenger—and how she responded to it. She then passes the ball to another person, who describes her passenger, and so on, until we've all had a turn.

Noticing Exercise (Aware)

Aim: To introduce and guide participants through the mindfulness of breath and body exercise, leaving enough time for an inquiry afterward.

Dialogue Example

Now, we are going to spend a few minutes getting present, just focusing on ourselves here and now.

Mindfulness of Breath and Body Exercise

I invite you to sit in a comfortable yet upright position in your chair, with your feet flat on the floor, arms and legs uncrossed, and hands resting in your lap. [Pause.] Let your eyes gently close, or fix them on a point in front of you. [Pause five seconds.]

Begin by gently bringing your attention to noticing your body. Start by directing your attention to your feet [pause]; notice the parts of your feet that are in contact with the ground. [Pause five seconds.] Notice the sensation of your shoes or socks on your feet. [Pause five seconds.] Then, bring your attention to noticing the sensation of sitting in the chair. [Pause.] See if you can notice the sense of your weight on the chair. [Pause five seconds.] Maybe notice parts of your body that are in contact with the chair [pause], and the parts of your body that don't contact the chair. [Pause five seconds.] If you drift off into your thoughts, simply acknowledge where your mind went and bring it back to noticing the sensation of sitting in the chair. [Pause five seconds.]

From time to time, you may notice that your attention has wandered off as you get caught up in your thoughts or other kinds of sensations. This is quite normal; it happens to everyone, and it may happen repeatedly. Each time you notice your mind wandering, take a split second to notice where it took you and gently bring your awareness back to noticing your body and the sense of your weight on the chair. [Pause five seconds.]

Next, direct your awareness to your breath. [Pause five seconds.] See if you can notice the sensation of breathing in [pause] and out [pause five seconds], allowing your stomach to expand, and your chest to gently rise and fall. [Pause five seconds.] Become aware of your breath flowing in and out of your body. Simply notice the natural flow of the breath, without changing or modifying it in any way. [Pause five seconds.]

Take a few slow, deep breaths. Notice the sensation of air filling your lungs as you breathe in and then deflating as you breathe out. [Pause five seconds.] You may notice the sensation of cool air around your nostrils as you inhale [pause], and the warm air as you exhale. [Pause five seconds.]

As you do this exercise, the feelings and sensations in your body may change. You may notice pleasant feelings or sensations, such as relaxation, calmness, or peacefulness. [Pause.] You may notice unpleasant feelings, such as boredom, frustration, or anxiety. [Pause.] Whatever feelings, urges, or sensations arise, whether pleasant or unpleasant, gently acknowledge their presence and let them be. Allow them to come and go, and keep your attention on your breath and the sensation of sitting in the chair. [Pause five seconds.]

Lastly, bring your attention back to noticing your breathing. [Pause five to ten seconds.] Notice again the steady rhythm of your breath that is with you all the time. [Pause five to ten seconds.] When you are ready, bring your attention back to the room. Open your eyes if they are closed. Notice what you can see [pause], and notice what you can hear. [Pause.] Push your feet into the ground and stretch and notice yourself stretching. Welcome back.

After completing the exercise, invite observations from participants. Ask about what they noticed and invite curiosity about their experience. Focus on drawing out differences between this experience and automatic-pilot experiences.

Dialogue Example

What did people notice when doing this exercise? Were you able to notice your body and the sensation of sitting in the chair? Did you notice your breath? Were people aware of their mind wandering off during the exercise? Were you able to bring your attention back to noticing your body and breath?

Passengers on the Bus Review

Aim: To remind participants about the key elements of the passengers on the bus metaphor, clarifying valued directions, the role of passengers, and our responses to passengers.

Dialogue Example

This metaphor is about the directions we want to go (our values) and the passengers who are on our bus and come along for the ride.

Before clarifying its key elements, first ask the group what they remember of the metaphor. If people need a reminder, show the animation, available at http://www.actforpsychosis.com. Here are the key elements of the metaphor:

- Life is like a journey, and you're the driver of your bus.

- You want to go to places and do what's important for you.

- On your bus there are many passengers.

- The passengers reflect your thoughts, feelings, and all kinds of inner states.

- Some are nice, but some are ugly, scary, and nasty.

- The scary ones threaten you and want to come up to the front of the bus where you'll see them.

- You take this very seriously and stop the bus (you don't go anywhere anymore) to struggle and fight with the passengers.

- You might try to avoid them, distract yourself from them, or throw them off the bus (but they are your inner states, so you can't get rid of them).

- You may also try to make a deal with them (if they'll keep quiet in the back of the bus, you'll do exactly what they tell you).

- This means your route plan is greatly impaired and you're always on guard when driving the bus.

- Now the passengers are in control of the bus. You, the driver, are not in control at all.

- Even though the passengers look scary, nasty, threatening, and so forth, they can't take control (unless you let them). They can't actually make you do something against your will.

Committed Action Review

Aim: To review the committed action exercise (driving license worksheets) participants completed at the end of last session, and to explore whether they have had the opportunity to increase openness responses.

Break into small groups with one facilitator to lead each group. Encourage participants to review the driving license worksheets they completed in the final workshop session. These highlighted committed actions they planned on taking between the workshops and booster sessions.

Encourage participants to describe how the committed actions went, whether they noticed any passengers or what they noticed about the process. Reinforce all efforts to take committed actions in valued directions, as well as any noticing on the part of participants. Reinforce all steps taken in or inclinations for valued directions, as these are part of building repertoires of effective behavior.

With those participants who had difficulty engaging in committed actions, reinforce any feedback they give in relation to thinking about taking action, such as small plans, inclinations, and so forth. Similarly, reinforce any noticing of barriers to doing the task, of struggling, and so on. This is a good opportunity to mention using defusion/acceptance and mindfulness skills when facing barriers, as well as the concept of openness to having unwanted experiences that are part of taking committed actions in valued directions.

Dialogue Example

We would like to hear how increasing your openness has gone since the last workshop session. What committed actions did you take? And what was that like?

What passengers did you notice? How did you respond to them? What did you do that let the passengers be while you moved in your valued direction?

After reviewing recent committed actions, the group should come together and review individual progress since the workshop ended. Write the following questions on the whiteboard, and ask participants to answer and discuss them:

- What was it like when you first came to the workshop?
- In the past, how did you deal with passengers?
- How do you deal with them now?
- What passengers have you noticed?
- How have you responded to them?
- How can you take these skills forward?

Dialogue Example

We are interested in hearing about your progress since the workshop.

Values Exercise

Aim: To give people an opportunity to further explore and connect with their values using values cards as prompts.

Break into small groups with one facilitator to lead each group. Each group should have a pack of values cards. Facilitators should encourage each participant to choose two cards he or she connects with. Then, participants should choose one card to talk about with their small group.

Facilitators could use this opportunity to encourage participants to identify ways they have noticed that person embodying that value, if they have. The facilitator should write these questions on the whiteboard:

- Why is this value important to you?
- What are you already doing to show this?

Dialogue Example

We would like you to have a look at the values cards and pick out two that really stand out for you—that you connect with. Then, choose one of the cards and answer the questions on the whiteboard in your head.

Skills Refresher

Aim: To give the group a chance to revisit some of the exercises covered in previous sessions.

Depending on what has been raised in the discussions in the session so far, on the whiteboard a facilitator should list the exercises in one of the three categories of open, aware, and active, and ask for a vote on which exercises participants would most like to review. Make sure you have all the exercises on hand so you can practice the most popular ones.

Aim to practice two exercises, using sessions 1 through 4 from this manual for instructions. If there is not enough time to cover all the exercises, plan to cover them in booster session 2. Here are examples of the exercises split into categories:

Open

- Passengers on the bus
- Committed action
- Pushing against the folder
- Having vs. buying into thoughts
- Sticky labels

Aware

- Noticing exercises: mindfulness of breath and body, mindful stretch, mindful walking, three-minute breathing space, mindful eating, leaves on the stream, clouds in the sky
- Identifying values, passengers, choices, and so forth
- Videos of Paul and George
- Facilitator phone call during the week
- Having vs. buying into thoughts
- Noticing others' values

Active

- Coming to the workshops
- Choosing valued directions
- SMART goals
- Committed actions during the week to move you closer to your goals or to move you in a valued direction
- Having vs. buying into thoughts
- Passengers on the bus

Committed Action (Active)

Aim: To set committed actions to be completed before the next session.

On the whiteboard write the following, to be done between now and the next booster session:

- Think of a value you identified during the four workshop sessions?
- What can you do during the next week in service of this value?
- What passengers might get in the way as you try to take this action?
- How might you respond to these passengers?

After reviewing the items on the whiteboard, have the group break into smaller groups, with a facilitator leading each one. Ask participants to complete the committed action worksheet to identify one values-based action they can take the following week that might move them toward their values. Remind people to set a SMART goal.

Within the small groups, facilitators should ask people if they would be willing to tell the others what they plan to do. Also, determine if participants would like one of the facilitators to contact them between sessions for a short five-minute phone call to discuss their committed actions. Make it clear that the phone calls are not designed as a way for the facilitator to check up on whether they have completed the action, but to serve as reminders of the process, such as mindful noticing and willingness.

Reinforce anything suggesting participants are willing to share their commitments with others. Ask participants to complete the developing aware skills worksheet, and see if they would be willing to practice one of the noticing exercises at least three times during the next week.

Dialogue Example

Think about the important value you identified using the values cards. Can you think of one action you could do over the next week that would reinforce that this is something important? Keep in mind that this is an opportunity to practice mindful noticing of passengers and your responses to them. If you complete the action, that's icing on the cake.

Closing the Session

Aim: To gather feedback from the group and reinforce the idea of attending the next booster session.

Come back together as a large group and ask for feedback about the workshop. Ask participants how they generally found the workshop and what they found most memorable. Reinforce the importance of attending the next booster session, and remind people of the dates.

To prompt feedback, consider writing the following on the whiteboard:

- How did you find the session today?
- What did you notice?
- What did you find helpful or unhelpful, or both?
- What was the most memorable thing from today's session?

If short on time, you could ask for "popcorn feedback": ask everyone to say one or two words to sum up what they found most memorable from the day's session.

Booster Session 2

The main purpose of booster session 2 is to review progress since the previous booster session; to support open, aware and, active skills; to review the content of the workshops; and to provide an opportunity to practice exercises. First, facilitators and participants will discuss what the workshops are about before doing a warm-up exercise. A facilitator will lead the group through the clouds in the sky exercise, followed by an inquiry debrief. The group will then break into small groups to review committed actions. After gathering together again as a large group, facilitators and participants will review open, aware, and active skills. The group will then act out the passengers on the bus metaphor, followed by a review of the workshop sessions and the closing of the session. The following session outline suggests an order for the topics and time frames. As always, the times given for each segment are approximate.

Timeline

Welcome and introduction	10 minutes
Noticing exercise (aware)	15 minutes
Committed action review	10 minutes
Skills refresher	45 minutes
Acting out the passengers on the bus exercise	25 minutes
Review of the workshop	10 minutes
Closing the session	5 minutes

Materials You'll Need

- Whiteboard

- Paper and pens
- Marker pens
- Refreshments

Additional Equipment for This Session

- A soft ball

Welcome and Introduction

Aim: To welcome participants to booster session 2 (of 2)—the final session—of the ACT for recovery workshop.

Remind people that the workshop will run for approximately two hours with a short break halfway through. If required, take care of housekeeping issues (e.g., location of fire escapes, bathrooms). Ask people again to wear name badges. Remind people of the purpose of the workshop by listing the following points on the whiteboard and reading through them:

- Developing life direction
- Increasing awareness of obstacles
- Learning the skills of open, aware, and active
- Connecting with each other and having fun

Dialogue Example

Just as a reminder, here are some of the key points we've covered over the course of these workshops.

After the review, help participants warm up for the session with a brief exercise. Invite everyone to stand up, and ask them to describe what passengers they noticed during the week and how they responded to them. Facilitators can start by giving their own examples.

Dialogue Example

To get us started, we'd like to invite you to do a short warm-up exercise. The person holding the ball briefly describes a value he has been working toward during the workshop. He then passes the ball to another person, who describes what value she has worked on, and so on, until we've all had a turn.

If participants are reluctant to talk about their own experiences, ask them if they noticed anyone else, such as friends or family members, working toward their values. Facilitators can volunteer their own values and what they have worked on.

Noticing Exercise (Aware)

Aim: To introduce and guide participants through the clouds in the sky exercise, leaving enough time for an inquiry afterward.

Dialogue Example

Now I'd like to invite you to do a noticing exercise. It will give you an idea of how we can be with and observe our unwanted thoughts and feelings, rather than struggle with them.

Clouds in the Sky Exercise

First, get in a comfortable position in your chair. Sit upright with your feet flat on the floor, your arms and legs uncrossed, and your hands resting on your lap. [Pause.] Allow your eyes to close, or fix them on a point in front of you. [Pause five seconds.] Take a couple of gentle breaths in and out. [Pause.] Notice the sensation of your own breath as you breathe in and out. [Pause five seconds.]

Now, try to imagine you are lying on a grassy hill on a warm spring day. [Pause.] Imagine feeling the ground beneath you [pause], the smell of the grass [pause], and the sounds of nearby trees blowing in the wind. [Pause five seconds.] Now, imagine you are looking up at the sky, watching clouds pass by. [Pause.] Start to become conscious of your thoughts and feelings. [Pause.] Each time a thought pops into your head, imagine placing it on one of these clouds and allowing it to float on by. [Pause.] If you think in words or images, place these on a cloud, and let them float by. [Pause five seconds.]

The goal is to continue watching the sky and to allow the clouds to keep moving by. [Pause.] Try not to change what shows up on the clouds in any way. If the clouds disappear or you go somewhere else mentally, just stop and notice this happening, and gently bring yourself back to watching the clouds in the sky. [Pause.]

If you have any thoughts or feelings about doing this exercise, place these on clouds as well. [Pause.] If your thoughts stop, just watch the sky and the clouds. Sooner or later your thoughts should start up again. [Pause five seconds.]

You are just observing each thought or feeling as a word or an image on a cloud. [Pause.] It is normal and natural to lose track of this exercise, and it will keep happening. When you notice yourself losing track, just bring yourself back to watching the clouds in the sky. [Pause.]

Let the clouds float at their own pace, and place any thought, feeling, sensation, or image that comes to mind on a cloud and allow it to float on by. [Pause five seconds.] When a thought hooks you, place that on a cloud and let it float by. [Pause.]

Finally, bring your attention back to your breathing. [Pause five seconds.] Notice again the steady rhythm of your breath that is with you all the time. [Pause five seconds.] Then, bring your awareness back to sitting in the chair, in this room. [Pause.] Gently open your eyes and notice what you can see. Push your feet onto the floor and have a stretch; notice yourself stretching. Welcome back.

After completing the exercise, invite observations from participants. Explore what people noticed in terms of their tendency to get hooked by thoughts and feelings and to bringing themselves back to observing the clouds.

Reinforce noticing, and draw participants' attention to how easily our minds can get hooked; stress that observing our experiences is a choice, and that it takes active noticing.

Some people may report that they wanted to hold on to positive thoughts rather than place them on clouds. While validating this response, emphasize that the aim is to observe the natural flow of thoughts, whether positive or negative, allowing them to come and go.

Dialogue Example

What did people notice while doing this exercise? What types of experiences hooked you? What was it like to let go of experiences so they could come and go without you holding on to them?

Committed Action Review

Aim: To review the committed action exercise participants completed at the end of last session, and to explore whether people have had the opportunity to increase openness responses.

On the whiteboard write the following:

- Think of the value you identified in the last session and the action linked to it.

- Did you notice any passengers show up in relation to this action?

- How did you experience the mindfulness practice during the week?

After reviewing the prompts, break into small groups with one facilitator to lead each group. Encourage participants to describe what passengers showed up or what they noticed about the process. Reinforce all efforts to take committed actions in valued directions, as well as any noticing on the part of participants. Reinforce all steps taken in or inclinations for valued directions, as these are part of building repertoires of effective behavior.

Dialogue Example

Toward the end of the previous session, we invited you to try to do something that was important to you, something that you valued. Did anyone have a go at this? What sorts of things did you notice?

How did the mindfulness practice go? Were you able to fit the practice into your usual routines? What did you notice?

Skills Refresher

Aim: To give the group a chance to revisit some of the exercises covered in previous sessions.

Depending on what has been raised in the discussions in the session so far, on the whiteboard a facilitator should list the exercises in the three categories of open, aware, and active, and ask for a vote on which exercises participants would most like to review. Make sure you have all the exercises on hand so you can practice the most popular ones. Here are examples of the exercises split into categories:

Open

- Passengers on the bus
- Committed action
- Pushing against the folder
- Having vs. buying into thoughts
- Sticky labels

Aware

- Noticing exercises: mindfulness of breath and body, mindful stretch, mindful walking, three-minute breathing space, mindful eating, leaves on the stream, clouds in the sky
- Identifying values, passengers, choices, and so forth
- Videos of Paul and George
- Facilitator phone call during the week
- Having vs. buying into thoughts
- Noticing others' values

Active

- Coming to the workshops
- Choosing valued directions
- SMART goals
- Committed actions during the week to move you closer to your goals or to move you in a valued direction
- Having vs. buying into thoughts
- Passengers on the bus

Acting Out the Passengers on the Bus Metaphor (Open)

Aim: To act out the passengers on the bus metaphor, ideally using content from a participant's example; otherwise you can make up an example or use Paul's or George's example from session 2. A video demonstration of the passengers on the bus exercise is available at http://www.actforpsychosis.com.

Explain to participants that you are going to be role-playing the passengers on the bus metaphor again, but this time you will ideally be using content from a participant's example. Participants will have the opportunity to try out being the driver and to try out three different responses to the passengers. Emphasize fun aspects of participating, but make it clear that it's okay to just observe the exercise.

Dialogue Example

Does anyone have an example they'd like to act out? [If nobody is forthcoming, the facilitator could ask:] Does anyone have an example they would be willing to direct someone else to act out?

If no one offers an example, act out a general example with common passengers—ones that participants reported in previous sessions. Or, use the example of being in and contributing to a group—a common experience for all participants!

Then ask for volunteers:

- **One person to act as the driver:** Have the driver decide on the main passengers he or she is struggling with.

- **Three to four people to act as passengers:** Ask for volunteers to play the roles of the driver's passengers. Provide them with a piece of paper with the name of their passenger on the front, and on the back write prompts of things each passenger might say so they can read them during the role-play.

- **One person to act as the valued direction:** Ask the driver to identify the valued direction that the passengers are getting in the way of. Summarize this in one or two words on a large sheet of paper, and ask for a volunteer to hold this representation of the driver's valued direction.

Fight/Struggle Scenario

In this scenario, have the driver role-play driving the bus (walking around the room with the passengers following) and stopping to fight and struggle (for example, yelling at passengers, arguing with them). Have the passengers behave like passengers (hassling, cajoling, pleading, distracting). Do this for two to four minutes. After the exercise, do the following:

- **Ask for feedback from the bus driver:** How was it to struggle with the passengers? (The facilitator can suggest that no matter how much one argues and fights with passengers, nothing changes the quality of stuckness.)

- **Ask for feedback from the passengers:** Did they feel in control of the driver?

- **Ask for feedback from the values representative:** Did this volunteer feel connected with the bus driver or ignored?

- **Ask for feedback from the wider group:** What did group members notice as observers?

Giving-In Scenario

Ask the driver to again drive the bus, this time role-playing *giving in* to the passengers (for example, agreeing with what they say, trying to make peace with passengers by allowing them to dictate where the bus goes, and so on). Do this for two to four minutes. After the exercise, do the following:

- **Ask for feedback from the bus driver:** How was it to give in to the passengers? What was it like to let go of the steering wheel? Did it feel like the passengers were in control of the bus's direction? Reinforce the qualities that it may feel better in the short term, but at the cost of important life areas—that is, being stuck in another way.

- **Ask for feedback from the passengers:** Did they feel in control of the driver?

- **Ask for feedback from the values representative:** Did this person feel connected to the bus driver or ignored?

- **Ask for feedback from the wider group:** What did they notice as observers?

Openness Scenario

Finally, ask the driver to practice an *openness* response (for example, using skills for noticing the passengers; thanking them for their comments; welcoming them on the bus; allowing them to be on the bus while steering it in a valued direction, with the passengers following behind saying or doing the things they usually say). Do this for two to four minutes. After the exercise, do the following:

- **Ask for feedback from the bus driver:** How was it to focus on values and keep them in mind while the passengers were saying or doing all those things?

- **Ask for feedback from the passengers:** Did they still feel in control of the driver?

- **Ask for feedback from the values representative:** Did this person feel connected to the bus driver or ignored?

- **Ask for feedback from the wider group:** What did group members notice as observers?

Debrief

Ask all participants how they experienced the exercise, and compare and contrast the three different scenarios. Highlight the differences between the first two responses and the openness (willingness) response in terms of key processes: present-moment focus, acceptance, defusion, values clarity, and committed action.

Review of the Workshop

Aim: To review the workshop with participants.

Ask participants about their experience attending the workshop and what they will take away from it. Write these questions on the whiteboard:

- What was your overall experience of the workshop?

- What have you noticed?

- How have you responded?

- What was it like for you when you came to the first workshop session?
- What's it like now?
- How can you take these skills forward?

Closing the Session

Aim: To bring the session to a close and gather feedback from the group about the ACT for recovery workshop.

Come back together as a large group and ask for feedback about the workshop. Ask participants about their general experience of the workshop and what they found most memorable. It's helpful to leave enough time for participants to say goodbye to each other and acknowledge the end of the workshop.

Dialogue Example

What was the most memorable thing about the workshop for each of you? What will you take away from it?

Acknowledgments

First, we would like to acknowledge all the client and caregiver participants, for their commitment in attending the workshops, and for their valuable feedback. We would also like to thank the peer-support cofacilitators, for their willingness to take on the cofacilitator role and for their openness during sessions, which has a positive impact on group cohesion and intervention delivery. We also acknowledge Guy's and St. Thomas' Charity and the Maudsley Charity, which funded the ACT for Life and ACT for Recovery evaluation studies, respectively.

We acknowledge our colleagues who assisted with the ACT for recovery manual, and with setting up and evaluating the groups. In particular, Suzanne Jolley, who led the ACT for Recovery study; Majella Byrne, who assisted with the manual; and research assistants Lucy Butler and Faye Sim. We also thank our chapter coauthors (Suzanne Jolley, Rumina Taylor, Georgina Bremner, and Natasha Avery) for their excellent contributions to this volume. A special thanks to our illustrator Kalos Chan for the great illustrations on our worksheets.

We would like to acknowledge the Association for Contextual Behavioral Science (ACBS) community and the people in the field who continue to inspire us to develop our practice in ACT and mindfulness. These include Kelly Wilson, Ross White, John Farhall, Yvonne Barnes-Holmes, Ciara McEnteggart, Joris Corthouts, and Neil Thomas. We have admired their work with people with psychosis and other mental health problems and have been very fortunate to work and collaborate with them. We would also like to thank our colleagues and friends in the area of cognitive behavioral therapy for psychosis, who have shaped our knowledge of developing, evaluating, and implementing psychological therapies for psychosis.

We would like to thank the ACBS Psychosis Special Interest Group for their support and work in bringing together ACT and CBS researchers and practitioners across the world. Through such cooperative efforts, our work becomes easier and more impactful.

We would particularly like to thank Steve Hayes. From the outset of the journey that led to this book, Steve has been there to encourage and motivate us, very generously providing his time and support, which has been invaluable.

It is important for us to acknowledge our colleagues and mentors in our places of work, including Emmanuelle Peters and Adrian Webster, who have nurtured and supported us over the years. Here, we must mention Suzanne Jolley again, who has enabled many of our clinical and academic achievements. She has provided us all with invaluable teaching, supervision, and management, for which we are incredibly grateful.

Last, but not least, we wish to acknowledge our respective friends and families for their ongoing love and support, which has allowed us to pursue our common value of making a positive difference in the lives of people with psychosis and their families.

APPENDIX A

Exercise Prompt Sheets

The following forms are available for download at http://www.actforpsychosis.com.

A1. Reservoir Metaphor

We all have "emotional reservoirs" of different types. Some supply energy, others supply health or well-being. When the reservoirs are full, we can maintain our energy or well-being, even in times of stress. If there is a drought, such as a bad day or week, or other forms of stress, we can maintain a healthy state because there is a supply in our reservoirs.

We know that sometimes being a caregiver can be difficult and challenging, and this can drain our reservoirs. If the reservoirs are dry, we can become vulnerable to stresses: there may be some energy or happiness, but only if daily events are going well. The combination of a dry reservoir and a bad day could be problematic and might lead to difficulties, such as an emotional crash, a lost temper, frustration, and so forth.

These workshops aim to teach you different ways of maintaining or replenishing your reservoirs so that you can maintain well-being and do more of what's important in life.

A2. Mindfulness of Breath and Body Exercise

I invite you to sit in a comfortable yet upright position in your chair, with your feet flat on the floor, arms and legs uncrossed, and hands resting in your lap. [Pause.] Let your eyes gently close, or fix them on a point in front of you. [Pause five seconds.]

Begin by gently bringing your attention to noticing your body. Start by directing your attention to your feet [pause]; notice the parts of your feet that are in contact with the ground. [Pause five seconds.] Notice the sensation of your shoes or socks on your feet. [Pause five seconds.] Then, bring your attention to noticing the sensation of sitting in the chair. [Pause.] See if you can notice the sense of your weight on the chair. [Pause five seconds.] Maybe notice parts of your body that are in contact with the chair [pause], and the parts of your body that don't contact the chair. [Pause five seconds.] If you drift off into your thoughts, simply acknowledge where your mind went and bring it back to noticing the sensation of sitting in the chair. [Pause five seconds.]

From time to time, you may notice that your attention has wandered off as you get caught up in your thoughts or other kinds of sensations. This is quite normal; it happens to everyone, and it may happen repeatedly. Each time you notice your mind wandering, take a split second to notice where it took you and gently bring your awareness back to noticing your body and the sense of your weight on the chair. [Pause five seconds.]

Next, direct your awareness to your breath. [Pause five seconds.] See if you can notice the sensation of breathing in [pause] and out [pause five seconds], allowing your stomach to expand, and your chest to gently rise and fall. [Pause five seconds.] Become aware of your breath flowing in and out of your body. Simply notice the natural flow of the breath, without changing or modifying it in any way. [Pause five seconds.]

Take a few slow, deep breaths. Notice the sensation of air filling your lungs as you breathe in and then deflating as you breathe out. [Pause five seconds.] You may notice the sensation of cool air around your nostrils as you inhale [pause], and the warm air as you exhale. [Pause five seconds.]

As you do this exercise, the feelings and sensations in your body may change. You may notice pleasant feelings or sensations, such as relaxation, calmness, or peacefulness. [Pause.] You may notice unpleasant feelings, such as boredom, frustration, or anxiety. [Pause.] Whatever feelings, urges, or sensations arise, whether pleasant or unpleasant, gently acknowledge their presence and let them be. Allow them to come and go, and keep your attention on your breath and the sensation of sitting in the chair. [Pause five seconds.]

Lastly, bring your attention back to noticing your breathing. [Pause five to ten seconds.] Notice again the steady rhythm of your breath that is with you all the time. [Pause five to ten seconds.] When you are ready, bring your attention back to the room. Open your eyes if they are closed. Notice what you can see [pause], and notice what you can hear. [Pause.] Push your feet into the ground and stretch and notice yourself stretching. Welcome back.

A3. Passengers on the Bus Metaphor

One way to think about barriers is to think about them as passengers on the bus of life.

Imagine life is like a journey, and you're the driver of your bus. You want to go places and do what's important for you. Over the course of your life, various passengers have boarded your bus. They reflect your thoughts, feelings, and all kinds of inner states. Some of them you like, such as happy memories or positive thoughts, and some you feel neutral about. And then there are passengers that you wish had not boarded the bus; they can be ugly, scary, and nasty.

So, you are driving your bus of life with all sorts of passengers on board. The scary passengers can threaten you and want to be at the front of the bus where you see them. You take this very seriously and stop the bus to struggle and fight with them. You may try to avoid them, distract yourself, or throw them off the bus, but they are your inner states, so you can't get rid of them. However, while the bus is stopped, you're not moving in the direction that's important to you.

You may also try to make deals with the passengers; you'll give in and do what they tell you to do if they agree to keep quiet in the back of the bus. This may feel a little easier than fighting with them, but it means the passengers are in control of the direction your bus is heading.

By fighting and struggling with the passengers or giving in to them, you, the driver, are not in control of your journey of life, and it's likely that you are not heading in a direction that is important to you. But what if, even though these passengers look scary, nasty, and threatening, they can't take control unless you allow them to? There can be different ways to respond to the passengers so that you can head in the direction that is important.

A4. Mindful Stretch Exercise

Begin by standing with your feet flat on the ground, hip-width apart. [Pause.] Notice how it feels to stand here [pause], noticing the sensations of the ground beneath your feet and the sensations in your body right now. Allow your shoulders to relax as best you can, and be present in your body. [Pause.] Start to bring your awareness to your breath and your stomach, being here, standing here, and breathing. [Pause five seconds.]

If you can, slowly begin to move your arms out to the side of your body. Gently allow your arms to move upward, bringing awareness to the environment around your arms, noticing whatever sensations are here as your arms rise. [Pause.] And gently bring the arms upward, slowly and mindfully until they're right up over your head, reaching for the sky. [Pause.]

Now, very gently, begin to move your arms over to the right so your body is slightly bending over. You might notice your hips moving slightly out to the left. [Pause.] Just notice whatever sensations you experience during this stretch. And, when you feel ready, move your arms back to center.

Next, allow your arms to move over to the left side. Your hips may move over to the right and your body very gently bends to the left. Just notice the sensations of the stretch. Then, very slowly, mindfully come back up to the center, and gently lower your arms to your sides. Notice whatever sensations that are here; notice any tendency for the arms to rush back to the side of your body. [Pause five seconds.]

When your arms reach your sides, just notice how your body is feeling right now. Notice any sensations of having done this stretch and being present, standing here with your feet on the ground, breathing and being aware of your breath. [Pause five seconds.]

Now, allow your hands to rest on your hips so your elbows are out to the sides. Settle into this posture, and, with your hips and feet still facing forward, very gently turn your upper body to the right. Keep your feet and hips facing forward, your upper body and shoulders moving to the right, just as far as they'll go. Not pushing anything, just gently twisting your body as far as it wants to be twisted right now. Then, gently, mindfully, come back to the center.

And now, gently twist your body to the left. Your feet steady on the ground, your hips facing forward, your shoulders and your upper body gently turned to the left as far as they will go. Then, gently coming back to the center, noticing the sensations of the stretch. Now, allow your arms to fall to the sides of your body. [Pause five seconds.]

Slowly move your head toward your right shoulder, gently stretching your neck just as far as it wants to go, noticing the sensation. Now, slowly come back to the center. Then, gently move your head to your left shoulder, mindfully stretching. Just noticing how your body feels right now. Then, bring your head back to the center and settle into this posture. [Pause five seconds.]

Come back to standing with your feet flat on the floor, your arms resting by your side, your shoulders back, your head straight, just resting here in this pose. Bring your awareness to your stomach and the rise and fall as you breathe in, and as you breathe out. Stand here in awareness, breathing, noticing how your body feels having done these stretches. [Pause.]

And, as this period of practice comes to an end, just rest here, and when you move away from this posture, see if you can bring mindfulness to your body as you move on into the day.

A5. Mindful Eating Exercise

We spend a lot of our lives not really being present in the here and now. Life can be busy and our minds can be easily distracted by our passengers. So now we are going to spend a few minutes focusing on the present by spending time noticing an object.

I'd like you to take the object you've been given and examine it. [Pause.]

Observe it with curiosity, as if you've never seen an object like this before. [Pause.]

Study its shape, its contours. [Pause five seconds.]

Notice its colors. Are there many different shades to it? [Pause five seconds.]

Notice the weight of it in your hand [pause], and the feel of it against your skin. [Pause.]

Run your fingers over the object and notice the way that the skin feels. [Pause.]

Raise it to your nose and smell it; really notice the aroma. [Pause.]

Break open the skin and notice what is inside. [Pause five seconds.]

Raise it to your nose again and see if there is a change in the aroma. [Pause.]

Notice the texture on the inside of the object. [Pause.]

Take out one segment of the object; hold it in your hand. [Pause.]

Feel the object between your fingers. [Pause.]

Take a moment to really study it. [Pause.]

Gently squeeze it and notice its texture. [Pause.]

Then, if you are willing, gently place the segment in your mouth. Don't chew it—just roll it around in your mouth. [Pause five seconds.]

Notice what's happening in your mouth; notice the salivation. [Pause.]

Notice the urge to bite. [Pause.]

When you are ready, bite into the object. Notice how it tastes. Notice the texture. [Pause five seconds.]

Slowly chew the object, and notice the sensations as you swallow it. [Pause.]

Appendix A: Exercise Prompt Sheets

[End by linking to values and purpose.] Even with a small object like this clementine, we can notice more by focusing on the present moment. Notice your experience of this object by being with it in this particular way. And now notice being here in the room, your purpose for coming here today, and the passengers that you carry with you while doing this.

A6. Paul's Story Transcript

I work in marketing, but it had got a bit stressful because the company was making people redundant at the same time as they were upping the workload. And I wasn't aware of how stressed I was getting, looking back, and I had to work really hard to concentrate. And I found that things were taking me twice as long as they used to, which was…it was really worrying, actually, and quite frustrating.

So, I just tried harder and I pushed on through, but my boss called me in because they could see that things weren't getting done, 'cause I had this particular problem with this project for a very important client. I forgot to do one whole aspect of the job and it had to be pointed out to me, so I found that really hard and embarrassing and quite upsetting actually.

And I couldn't really say anything to anyone. And it was after a particularly hard meeting with them, I took a phone call at my desk. I can't remember who that was from actually. Anyway, it doesn't matter. So I heard this clicking noise on the line and I hadn't heard that before. And then it kept happening. So I realized that they were recording my conversations, and the more I thought about it, the more I realized that they were watching me on CCTV, and they were checking my emails.

And I asked others in the office if they could hear clicking on their phones, and I even asked a few of them if they could hear it on my phone, but it never happened when I handed somebody the phone. It just stopped. So, it was like they were watching me doing it.

So I started to feel really unsafe at work, and I thought, *Well, why don't I just take work home, 'cause then they couldn't record me or watch me.* And I worked evenings and weekends, and I worked really hard to catch up, but it didn't seem to make any difference.

And I was really tired as I was finding it difficult to sleep and keep up with everything. I even approached my bosses, and I told them that I knew what they were doing, but of course they denied it to my face.

And I told my fiancé, Jane, and we discussed it a lot, but in the end she just thought I was imagining it, and she got totally fed up with me going on and on and on about it. And in the end she ended up leaving me. That was really hard. I thought she understood because she knew about my difficulties years ago. We were gonna get married next year, and we were talking about starting a family, but now, well, that's all gone.

So anyway, things reached a head and my Mum took me to the GP because I wasn't eating or sleeping at that point, and she was worried about me because of what's happened in the past. And when I saw the doctor, she signed me off on sick leave, and that meant reduced pay, although it had an upside because it meant that they couldn't sack me.

So, with Jane gone, I couldn't keep up with the rent, so Mum said that I could live with them, which was really nice of them, but I'm thirty-four, and to be living back with my parents was just really hard.

I felt like a real burden. Don't get me wrong, Mum's great, but we started having a few arguments because she kept trying to make me eat 'cause I was worried about my food. Unless it was properly packaged, how did I know that somebody hadn't tampered with it? And it's not that I didn't trust Mum, but how do I know it's not been messed with before it's reached the house?

I was okay with food in sealed packages 'cause they couldn't be messed with, but I wasn't eating brilliantly. Mum was really worried 'cause I seemed to have lost a lot of weight and I was feeling really, really anxious pretty much most of the time. I hated that feeling. I would end up avoiding all sorts of situations that made me feel that way.

I can remember thinking *I'm going crazy*, and that all my friends knew. So I stopped seeing my friends, which made me feel better for a bit because I didn't want them to see me like that, but it got really lonely. But I'm feeling a bit better now, and I'm seeing my care coordinator regularly, and although I'm still off sick from work, I'm starting to think about going back part-time.

Anyway, at the moment I'm just focusing on getting better day to day.

A7. George's Story Transcript

My son Paul was originally diagnosed with psychosis when he was at university. And I think the whole thing was triggered by stress and some rather misplaced cannabis use, but then he's genetically hardwired for it because my father had schizophrenia, or at least that's what we were finally told. And so, with the added pressure of university, something in his head just…went.

I still feel very terrible about that whole episode. Not only did I pass on genes, but I also had to give the doctor's permission to section him. It's an awful thing to have to do for and to your child. I hope he's forgiven me. We don't tend to talk about it. But then we didn't know what to do or how to help him. He's always been a high achiever. We encourage both our children to work hard and get somewhere in life. If you want to achieve things, then you have to work hard and put the effort in. And that's how we brought them both up.

Although I do sometimes wonder if this is all part of the picture of what caused him to get ill. But what can you do? You don't encourage your kids and people think you don't care. It's very difficult as a parent.

Anyway, Paul came home a few months ago, and he was convinced that his bosses wanted to sack him and that they were watching and monitoring his every move. He constantly talked about it. He was so worried that he'd take work home and be up all hours. He even confronted one of his bosses!

He was signed off on sick leave, but he continued to work well into the night. I just didn't know what to do. He's my son, and I love him and I want to support him. Everything started to go wrong when his fiancé upped and left, 'cause she couldn't take it anymore. Paul was on reduced pay from work and couldn't afford to keep his place, so he moved back in with his Mum and me.

I had to do lots for him at the time, but he's my son and I wanted to help him, but it was a bit like having a young child to look after. He needed me.

Jean, my wife, didn't agree. She thought I was doing way too much for him. It's one of the things we started arguing about. I didn't feel particularly supported by her at the time. She couldn't see that Paul needed the help, that he was unwell.

Lee, his brother, was no better. He could've done more for his brother, but he just buried his head in the sand. I wish he'd seen him more. They used to be really close as children.

This food and eating thing really got me down. He got it into his head that people were trying to tamper with his food, and he wouldn't eat anything fresh that had been cooked by someone else. He'd eat prepackaged meals, which I'd bought more of just to get some food down him. He was getting so thin. But it was so expensive.

I felt so guilty that I'd passed this on to him, and I started to wonder if it was my parenting that caused him to be unwell. I suppose I did more for him as a way of compensating for how bad I felt. Jean just got really angry with me. She said that I was spoiling Paul.

I found it all really hard, to be honest. I remember thinking I was a hopeless father. I sort of gave up at one point and just believed it. Felt like my life was on hold. I put everything into caring for Paul because I'm his dad and I want him to be healthy and have a good life, but it was at the cost of mine it seemed.

I had to take quite a lot of time off work, and I felt awful that my colleagues had to pick up the slack for me. I think my boss was starting to lose patience. I used to play football once a week, and I started to miss that. I didn't see my friends 'cause I didn't like leaving Paul on his own. I also didn't really want to discuss our private business with anyone. I wouldn't want Paul's problems becoming common knowledge. I wouldn't want people judging us; life's hard enough.

But then I felt the only way I could relax was to have a whiskey, but then the one turned into two, and then several more! I found it easier to deal with things once I was a bit drunk, and it certainly helped me to get to sleep. But soon I was drinking every day; I just wanted to escape. I didn't want to have to deal with Paul, and I knew Jean would just be angry with me. I think I actually started to resent Paul a bit, but that made me feel awful and like a bad father.

But, thankfully, things have got a bit better. Paul's meeting with his care coordinator regularly, and he's starting to eat and sleep properly again. He's still living with us, but he wants to return to work, and I can see him becoming more like his old self.

I just wish I could protect him from this happening again.

A8. Pushing Against the Folder Exercise

I invite you to take your folder in both hands. I want you to imagine this folder represents all the difficult thoughts, feelings, memories, and sensations you've been struggling with for so long. And I'd like you to take hold of your folder and grip it as tightly as you can. [Pause.]

Now, I'd like you to hold your folder up in front of your face so you can't see me anymore—bring it up so close to your face that it almost touches your nose. Imagine that this is what it's like to be completely caught up with these thoughts, feelings, or memories.

Now, just notice. What's it like trying to have a conversation or to connect with me while you're all caught up in your thoughts and feelings? Do you feel connected with me, or engaged with me? Are you able to read the expressions on my face? See what I'm doing?

And what's your view of the room like, while you're all caught up in this stuff? [Pause.]

So, while you're completely absorbed in all this stuff, you're missing out on a lot. You're disconnected from the world around you, and you're disconnected from me. Notice, too, that while you're holding on tightly to this stuff, you can't do the things that make your life work. Check it out—grip the folder as tightly as you possibly can.

Can you really connect with loved ones while you're caught up with this stuff? Can you do your job properly?

Now, without letting go of your folder, I want you to try and push it away. Try to get rid of all those difficult thoughts and feelings.

Keep pushing. You can't stand these feelings; you want them to go away; push harder.

Notice how much effort and energy it requires trying to make these thoughts and feelings go away. [Pause.]

So here you are, trying very hard to push away all these painful thoughts and feelings. You've probably tried distracting yourself with TV, music, computers, drink, avoiding people, avoiding work, so forth, and so on.

You've been doing this for years, just pushing and pushing. Are those painful thoughts and feelings going anywhere? [Pause.]

You're able to keep them at arm's length, but what's the cost to you? How does it feel in your shoulders?

While you are doing this, pushing your folder away, would you be able to connect with your friends and family, cook dinner, do your job effectively, or drive your bus of life? Do you think it would be easy to have a conversation and really connect with the other person while you're doing this? [Pause.]

So, trying to push all those feelings away is eating up a lot of effort and energy. This is what you've been doing for so long now, trying to get rid of unpleasant thoughts and feelings. And yet, they keep showing up; they are still having an effect on your life.

Now, rest the folder on your lap for a moment. Just let these thoughts and feelings sit there on your lap. [Pause five seconds.]

How does that feel? Isn't it a lot less effort?

Those painful, distracting thoughts and feelings are still there. But notice the difference: now you can hug someone you love, cook dinner, or drive your bus of life. It's not draining you or tiring you out. [Pause.]

Isn't that easier than constantly trying to push these feelings away or being so caught up with them? [Mime pushing the folder away and holding it up to your nose.]

The difficult feelings are still there. And, of course, you don't want them; who would want all these painful thoughts and feelings? But notice how this stuff is having much less of an impact on you. Now I'm sure in the ideal world you'd like to do this [mime throwing the folder on the floor].

But here's the thing: you've been trying to do that for years. You've clearly put a lot of time, effort, and money into trying to get rid of these thoughts and feelings. And yet, despite all that effort, they're still showing up. They're still here today.

One of the goals of these workshops is to teach you how to be open to experiencing difficult thoughts and feelings instead of fighting with them or trying to avoid them.

A9. Acting Out the Passengers on the Bus Exercise

To begin this exercise, ask for volunteers:

- **One person needs to act as the driver (either Paul or George).** Have the group decide on the main passengers (for example, worry, paranoia, guilt, and so forth; thoughts like *I'm going crazy* or *I'm a bad father*) based on content from the video vignette.

- **Another three to four people need to act as passengers.** Ask for volunteers to play the role of the driver's passengers. Provide them with sticky notes with the label of their passenger, and remind them of the kinds of things each passenger would say (for example, Paul's "worry" passenger might talk about people recording him or trying to poison his food; George's "guilty" passenger might talk about him being a bad father who passed on his genes).

- **One person needs to act as the valued direction.** Ask the driver to identify the valued direction that the passengers are getting in the way of. Summarize this in one or two words on a large sheet of paper, and ask for a volunteer to hold this representation of the driver's valued direction.

Fight/Struggle Scenario

In this scenario, have the driver role-play driving the bus (walking around the room with the passengers following) and stopping to fight and struggle (for example, yelling at passengers, arguing with them). Have the passengers behave like passengers (hassling, cajoling, pleading, distracting). Do this for two to four minutes. After the exercise, do the following:

- **Ask for feedback from the bus driver:** How was it to struggle with the passengers? (The facilitator can suggest that no matter how much one argues and fights with passengers, nothing changes the quality of stuckness.)

- **Ask for feedback from the passengers:** Did they feel in control of the driver?

- **Ask for feedback from the values representative:** Did this volunteer feel connected with the bus driver or ignored?

- **Ask for feedback from the wider group:** What did group members notice as observers?

Giving-In Scenario

Ask the driver to again drive the bus, this time role-playing *giving in* to the passengers (for example, agreeing with what they say, trying to make peace with passengers by allowing them to dictate where the bus goes, and so on). Do this for two to four minutes. After the exercise, do the following:

- **Ask for feedback from the bus driver:** How was it to give in to the passengers? What was it like to let go of the steering wheel? Did it feel like the passengers were in control of the bus's direction? Reinforce the qualities that it may feel better in the short term, but at the cost of important life areas—that is, being stuck in another way.

- **Ask for feedback from the passengers:** Did they feel in control of the driver?

- **Ask for feedback from the values representative:** Did this person feel connected to the bus driver or ignored?

- **Ask for feedback from the wider group:** What did group members notice as observers?

Openness Scenario

Finally, ask the driver to practice an *openness* response (for example, using skills for noticing the passengers; thanking them for their comments; welcoming them on the bus; allowing them to be on the bus while steering it in a valued direction, with the passengers following behind saying or doing the things they usually say). Do this for two to four minutes. After the exercise, do the following:

- **Ask for feedback from the bus driver:** How was it to focus on your values and keep them in mind while the passengers were saying or doing all those things?

- **Ask for feedback from the passengers:** Did they still feel in control of the driver?

- **Ask for feedback from the values representative:** Did this person feel connected to the bus driver or ignored?

- **Ask for feedback from the wider group:** What did group members notice as observers?

A10. Three-Minute Breathing Space Exercise

Now we're going to practice a short breathing exercise that may allow you to step out of automatic mode and reconnect with the present moment.

Find a comfortable, upright position, and either close your eyes or focus on a spot in front of you. Now take a deep breath to bring yourself into the present moment [pause], just noticing whatever you are experiencing right now. Notice any sensations, be they of discomfort or tension. Notice your feet on the ground, or, if you're sitting, notice whatever you are sitting on; notice your clothes against your body and the air against the skin. [Pause five seconds.]

And now, notice whatever is in your mind. Whatever thoughts are here, and as best you can, just observe your thoughts as they are in your mind right now. [Pause.] Now notice whatever you are feeling emotionally. Don't try to change it, but just notice how you are feeling. [Pause five seconds.]

And now, bring your attention to your breath, just noticing the rise and fall of your stomach as you breathe in [pause], and as you breathe out. [Pause five seconds.] Notice the cool air flowing in through your nose as you inhale and the warm air as you exhale [pause], as you breathe in and out. [Pause.]

If you find your mind wandering away from your breath, simply bring it back to noticing each breath in, and out, as they follow, one after the other. [Pause five seconds.]

And now, allow your awareness to expand to encompass your breath moving in your body [pause], bringing your awareness to your thinking [pause], and whatever you are feeling emotionally right now. Gently broaden this awareness to notice the whole experience, holding everything in awareness. [Pause five seconds.]

Now bring your attention back to the room; open your eyes if they are closed. Notice what you can see; notice what you can hear. Push your feet into the ground and have a stretch; notice yourself stretching. Welcome back!

A11. Leaves on the Stream Exercise

I invite you to sit in a comfortable yet upright position in your chair, with your feet flat on the floor, your arms and legs uncrossed, and your hands resting in your lap. [Pause.] Let your eyes gently close, or fix them on a point in front of you. [Pause five seconds.] Take a couple of gentle breaths in [pause], and out. [Pause.] Notice the sound and feel of your own breath as you breathe in [pause], and out. [Pause five seconds.]

Now, I'd like you to imagine that you are standing by the bank of a gently flowing stream watching the water flow. [Pause.] Imagine feeling the ground beneath you, the sounds of the water flowing past, and the way the stream looks as you watch it. [Pause five seconds.] Imagine that there are leaves from trees, of all different shapes, sizes, and colors, floating past on the stream and you are just watching these float on the stream. This is all you need to do for the time being. [Pause five seconds.]

Start to become aware of your thoughts, feelings, or sensations. [Pause.] Each time you notice a thought, feeling, or sensation, imagine placing it on a leaf and letting it float down the stream. [Pause five seconds.] Do this regardless of whether the thoughts, feelings, or sensations are positive or negative, pleasurable or painful. [Pause.] Even if they are the most wonderful thoughts, place them on a leaf and let them float by. [Pause five seconds.]

If your thoughts stop, just watch the stream. Sooner or later your thoughts should start up again. [Pause five seconds.] Allow the stream to flow at its own rate. [Pause.] Notice any urges to speed up or slow down the stream, and let these be on leaves as well. Let the stream flow how it will. [Pause five seconds.]

If you have thoughts, feelings, or sensations about doing this exercise, place these on leaves as well. [Pause five seconds.]

If a leaf gets stuck or won't go away, let it hang around. For a little while, all you are doing is observing this experience; there is no need to force the leaf down the stream. [Pause five seconds.]

If you find yourself getting caught up with a thought or feeling, such as boredom or impatience, simply acknowledge it. Say to yourself, "Here's a feeling of boredom," or "Here's a feeling of impatience." Then place those words on a leaf, and let them float on by. [Pause five seconds.]

You are just observing each experience and placing it on a leaf on the stream. It is normal and natural to lose track of this exercise, and it will keep happening. When you notice yourself losing track, just bring yourself back to watching the leaves on the stream. [Pause ten seconds.]

Notice the stream, and place any thoughts, feelings, or sensations on the leaves and let them gently float down the stream. [Pause five seconds.]

Finally, allow the image of the stream to dissolve, and slowly bring your attention back to sitting in the chair, in this room. [Pause.] Gently open your eyes and notice what you can see. Notice what you can hear. Push your feet into the floor and have a stretch. Notice yourself stretching. Welcome back.

A12. Mindful Walking Exercise

Start by standing with your feet flat on the ground, and bring your attention to the soles of your feet. [Pause.] Wiggle your toes if this helps to focus your awareness. [Pause.] Start to become aware of your weight passing through the soles of your feet into the ground. Notice all the delicate movements that happen in order to keep us balanced and upright. [Pause.]

Now, start walking at a slow pace. Try not to change the way you walk; simply be aware of the way you are walking. [Pause.] Your body may do a funny wobble as soon as you become aware of yourself. Don't worry, that's a natural effect. [Pause five seconds.]

Direct your attention to the soles of your feet, being aware of the constant patterns of landing and lifting. [Pause five seconds.] Be aware of your foot as the heel first contacts the ground. Notice how your foot rolls forward onto the ball, and then lifts and travels through the air again. [Pause.] Visualize your feet going through this pattern as you walk. [Pause five seconds.]

Try to be aware of all the different sensations in your feet [pause], not just the contact with the soles of your feet but the connection between the toes [pause], and the sensation of your feet against the fabric of your socks or shoes. [Pause.] Try to let your feet be as relaxed as possible. [Pause five seconds.]

Now, direct your attention to your ankles. [Pause.] Notice the sensation in your joints. Allow your ankles to be relaxed. Try not to resist the movement of your ankles in any way. Now, become aware of your lower legs [pause], your shins [pause], and your calves as you walk. [Pause five seconds.]

You might notice that your mind wanders while doing this exercise. This is common, and it may happen again and again. If it does, try to bring your attention back to the exercise of walking and focusing on your body. [Pause five seconds.]

Now, expand your awareness to your thighs [pause]; notice how your clothing feels on your skin. [Pause.] Be aware of the front and rear thigh muscles. [Pause.] Become aware of the whole of your pelvis [pause], and notice all the movements that are going on in your pelvis as you walk. Notice how one hip moves forward, and then the other [pause]; one hip lifts, the other sinks, and you walk. [Pause.] Just keep walking and noticing your body as you do this exercise. [Pause five seconds.]

Next, notice your shoulders. [Pause.] Try to see how they are moving in rhythm as you walk. [Pause.] Are they moving opposite to your hips? Are your arms simply hanging by your sides and swinging naturally? [Pause five seconds.]

Lastly, come to a natural stop and just experience yourself standing. [Pause.] Notice what it's like to no longer be mobile. [Pause five seconds.] Notice once more the balancing act that's going on to keep you upright. [Pause.] Feel once again the weight traveling down through the soles of your feet into the ground. Congratulate yourself for your intention to practice mindful walking, no matter how many times your mind was pulled away from the walk, or how "well" you thought your practice went today. Just notice that the intention to be mindful is the key to practice. Welcome back.

A13. Key Messages Cards

Open		
Passengers on the Bus Exercise	Committed Actions	Pushing Against the Folder Exercise
Having vs. Buying into Thoughts Exercise	Sticky Labels Exercise	

Aware		
Mindfulness of Breath and Body Exercise	Mindful Stretch Exercise	Mindful Eating Exercise
Three-Minute Breathing Space Exercise	Leaves on the Stream Exercise	Mindful Walking Exercise
Clouds in the Sky Exercise	Videos of Paul and George	Weekly Telephone Call from Facilitator
Having vs. Buying into Thoughts Exercise	Noticing Others' Values Exercise	

Active		
Coming to the Workshops	Choosing Valued Directions	SMART Goals
Committed Action	Having vs. Buying into Thoughts Exercise	Passengers on the Bus Exercise

A14. Clouds in the Sky Exercise

First, get in a comfortable position in your chair. Sit upright with your feet flat on the floor, your arms and legs uncrossed, and your hands resting on your lap. [Pause.] Allow your eyes to close, or fix them on a point in front of you. [Pause five seconds.] Take a couple of gentle breaths in and out. [Pause.] Notice the sensation of your own breath as you breathe in and out. [Pause five seconds.]

Now, try to imagine you are lying on a grassy hill on a warm spring day. [Pause.] Imagine feeling the ground beneath you [pause], the smell of the grass [pause], and the sounds of nearby trees blowing in the wind. [Pause five seconds.] Now, imagine you are looking up at the sky, watching clouds pass by. [Pause.] Start to become conscious of your thoughts and feelings. [Pause.] Each time a thought pops into your head, imagine placing it on one of these clouds and allowing it to float on by. [Pause.] If you think in words or images, place these on a cloud, and let them float by. [Pause five seconds.]

The goal is to continue watching the sky and to allow the clouds to keep moving by. [Pause.] Try not to change what shows up on the clouds in any way. If the clouds disappear or you go somewhere else mentally, just stop and notice this happening, and gently bring yourself back to watching the clouds in the sky. [Pause.]

If you have any thoughts or feelings about doing this exercise, place these on clouds as well. [Pause.] If your thoughts stop, just watch the sky and the clouds. Sooner or later your thoughts should start up again. [Pause five seconds.]

You are just observing each thought or feeling as a word or an image on a cloud. [Pause.] It is normal and natural to lose track of this exercise, and it will keep happening. When you notice yourself losing track, just bring yourself back to watching the clouds in the sky. [Pause.]

Let the clouds float at their own pace, and place any thought, feeling, sensation, or image that comes to mind on a cloud and allow it to float on by. [Pause five seconds.] When a thought hooks you, place that on a cloud and let it float by. [Pause.]

Finally, bring your attention back to your breathing. [Pause five seconds.] Notice again the steady rhythm of your breath that is with you all the time. [Pause five seconds.] Then, bring your awareness back to sitting in the chair, in this room. [Pause.] Gently open your eyes and notice what you can see. Push your feet onto the floor and have a stretch; notice yourself stretching. Welcome back.

A15. Client Satisfaction Questionnaire

Please help us improve future workshops by answering some questions about the ACT for recovery workshop. We are interested in your honest opinions, whether they are positive or negative. *Please answer all the questions.* We also welcome your comments and suggestions. Thank you very much. We appreciate your help.

Q1	Excellent	Good	Fair	Poor
How would you rate the quality of the workshops you have attended?	4	3	2	1
Q2	No, definitely not.	No, not really.	Maybe.	Yes, definitely.
Have you been able to take something from the workshops and use it in your life?	1	2	3	4
Q3	Yes, they helped a great deal.	Yes, they helped somewhat.	No, they didn't really help.	No, they seemed to make things worse.
Have the workshops helped you deal more effectively with your problems?	4	3	2	1
Q4	Very satisfied	Mostly satisfied	Indifferent or mildly dissatisfied	Quite dissatisfied
In an overall, general sense, how satisfied are you with the workshops?	4	3	2	1

Q5	Quite dissatisfied	Indifferent or mildly dissatisfied	Mostly satisfied	Very satisfied
How satisfied are you with the therapists running the workshops?	1	2	3	4
Q6	No, definitely not.	No, I don't think so.	Yes, I think so.	Yes, definitely.
Would you come back to a workshop like this again?	1	2	3	4
Q7	No, definitely not.	No, I don't think so.	Yes, I think so.	Yes, definitely.
Did the workshops help you find out what is important to you?	1	2	3	4
Q8	No, definitely not.	No, I don't think so.	Yes, I think so.	Yes, definitely.
If a friend or someone you knew needed similar help, would you recommend the workshops to him or her?	1	2	3	4

Please complete the following statements:

The things I liked best about the workshops were:

The things I liked least were:

If I could change one thing about the workshops it would be:

Any further comments:

A16. The ACTs of ACT Fidelity Measure

Workshop session number: _____ Date: _____

For the workshop session, please rate for the presence of each of the components below.

For each component that is *present*, please rate how appropriate it is for this stage of therapy, and then rate group responsiveness to this component.

ACT therapeutic stance	*How present in this session?*	*How appropriate for this session?*	*Group responsiveness?*
	0 = Not at all 1 = Minimal 2 = Satisfactory 3 = High 4 = Very high	0 = Inappropriate 1 = Minimally 2 = Satisfactory 3 = Highly 4 = Very high	0 = Unresponsive 1 = Minimal 2 = Satisfactory 3 = High 4 = Very high
Developing acceptance and willingness/undermining experiential control	*How present in this session?*	*How appropriate for this session?*	*Group responsiveness?*
	0 = Not at all 1 = Minimal 2 = Satisfactory 3 = High 4 = Very high	0 = Inappropriate 1 = Minimally 2 = Satisfactory 3 = Highly 4 = Very high	0 = Unresponsive 1 = Minimal 2 = Satisfactory 3 = High 4 = Very high
Undermining cognitive fusion	*How present in this session?*	*How appropriate for this session?*	*Group responsiveness?*
	0 = Not at all 1 = Minimal 2 = Satisfactory 3 = High 4 = Very high	0 = Inappropriate 1 = Minimally 2 = Satisfactory 3 = Highly 4 = Very high	0 = Unresponsive 1 = Minimal 2 = Satisfactory 3 = High 4 = Very high
Getting in contact with the present moment	*How present in this session?*	*How appropriate for this session?*	*Group responsiveness?*
	0 = Not at all 1 = Minimal 2 = Satisfactory 3 = High 4 = Very high	0 = Inappropriate 1 = Minimally 2 = Satisfactory 3 = Highly 4 = Very high	0 = Unresponsive 1 = Minimal 2 = Satisfactory 3 = High 4 = Very high

Distinguishing the conceptualized self from self-as-context	How present in this session?	How appropriate for this session?	Group responsiveness?
	0 = Not at all 1 = Minimal 2 = Satisfactory 3 = High 4 = Very high	0 = Inappropriate 1 = Minimally 2 = Satisfactory 3 = Highly 4 = Very high	0 = Unresponsive 1 = Minimal 2 = Satisfactory 3 = High 4 = Very high
Defining valued directions	How present in this session?	How appropriate for this session?	Group responsiveness?
	0 = Not at all 1 = Minimal 2 = Satisfactory 3 = High 4 = Very high	0 = Inappropriate 1 = Minimally 2 = Satisfactory 3 = Highly 4 = Very high	0 = Unresponsive 1 = Minimal 2 = Satisfactory 3 = High 4 = Very high
Building patterns of committed action	How present in this session?	How appropriate for this session?	Group responsiveness?
	0 = Not at all 1 = Minimal 2 = Satisfactory 3 = High 4 = Very high	0 = Inappropriate 1 = Minimally 2 = Satisfactory 3 = Highly 4 = Very high	0 = Unresponsive 1 = Minimal 2 = Satisfactory 3 = High 4 = Very high

ACT-Inconsistent Techniques/Proscribed Behaviors	How Present in This Session?
Did the facilitator explain the "meaning" of paradoxes or metaphors (possibly to develop "insight")?	0 = Not at all 1 = Minimal 2 = Moderate 3 = High 4 = Very high
Did the facilitator engage in criticism, judgment, or taking a "one-up" position?	0 = Not at all 1 = Minimal 2 = Moderate 3 = High 4 = Very high

Did the facilitator argue with, lecture, coerce, or attempt to convince the participant?	0 = Not at all 1 = Minimal 2 = Moderate 3 = High 4 = Very high
Did the facilitator substitute his or her opinions for the participant's genuine experience of what is working or not working?	0 = Not at all 1 = Minimal 2 = Moderate 3 = High 4 = Very high
Did the facilitator model the need to resolve contradictory or difficult ideas, feelings, memories, and the like?	0 = Not at all 1 = Minimal 2 = Moderate 3 = High 4 = Very high
Evidence for delusional beliefs: Did the facilitator assess the evidence the participant uses to support his or her delusional beliefs?	0 = Not at all 1 = Minimal 2 = Moderate 3 = High 4 = Very high
Validity testing/behavioral experiments: Did the facilitator encourage the participant to (1) engage in specific behaviors for the purpose of testing the validity of his or her beliefs, or (2) make explicit predictions about external events so that the outcomes of those events could serve as tests of those predictions, or (3) review the outcome of previous validity tests?	0 = Not at all 1 = Minimal 2 = Moderate 3 = High 4 = Very high
Verbal challenge of delusions: Did the facilitator challenge the participant's beliefs through discussion?	0 = Not at all 1 = Minimal 2 = Moderate 3 = High 4 = Very high

Overall Rating

How would you rate the facilitator's performance *overall* in leading group ACT in this session?

0	1	2	3	4	5	6
Poor	Barely adequate	Mediocre	Satisfactory	Good	Very good	Excellent

APPENDIX B

Session Worksheets

The following forms are available for download at http://www.actforpsychosis.com.

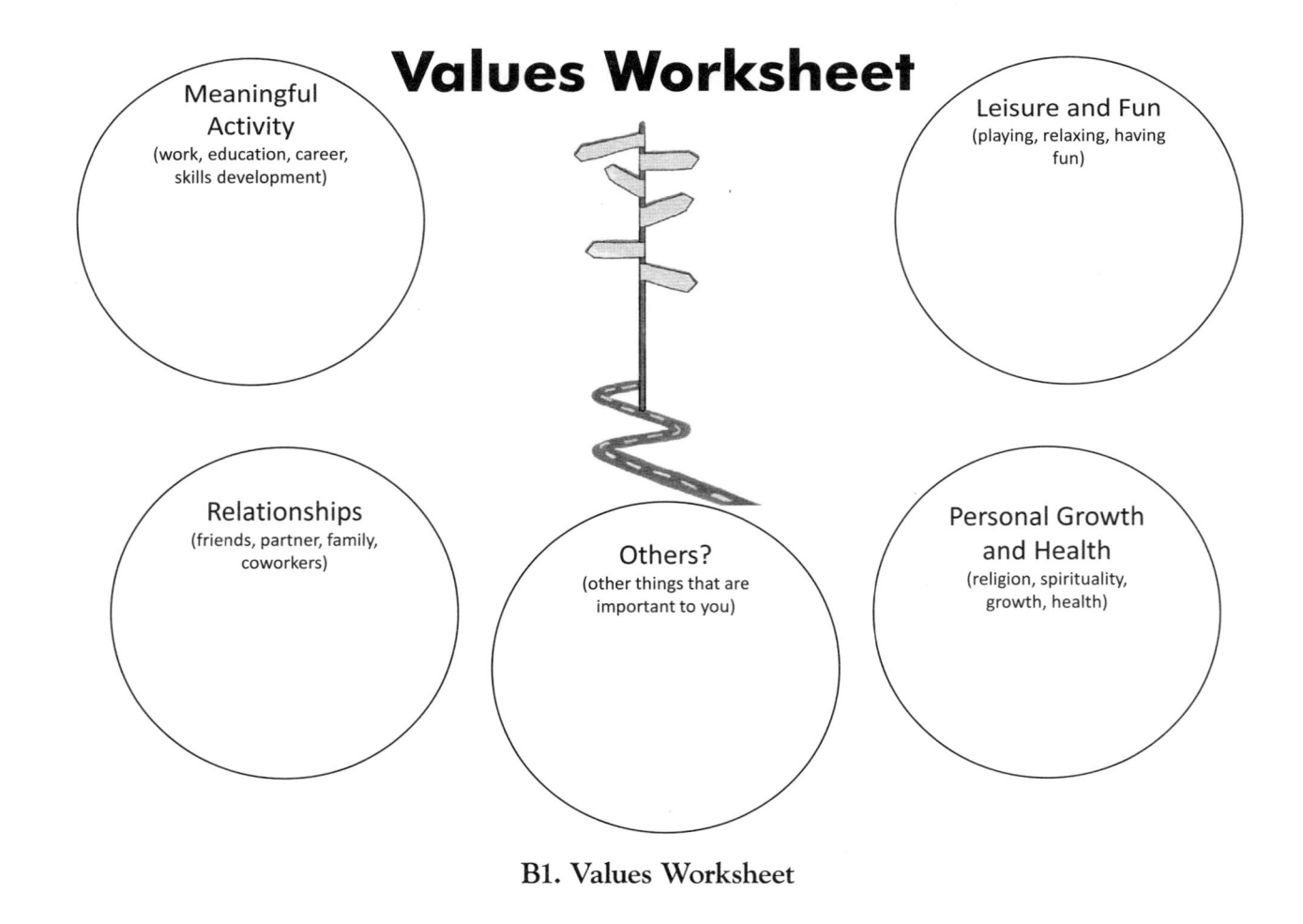

ACT for Psychosis Recovery

Values Worksheet

- **Leisure and Fun** (playing, relaxing, having fun)
- **Personal Growth and Health** (religion, spirituality, growth, health)
- **Others?** (other things that are important to you)
- **Meaningful Activity** (work, education, career, skills development)
- **Relationships** (friends, partner, family, coworkers)

B1. Values Worksheet

Appendix B: Session Worksheets

Passengers on the Bus

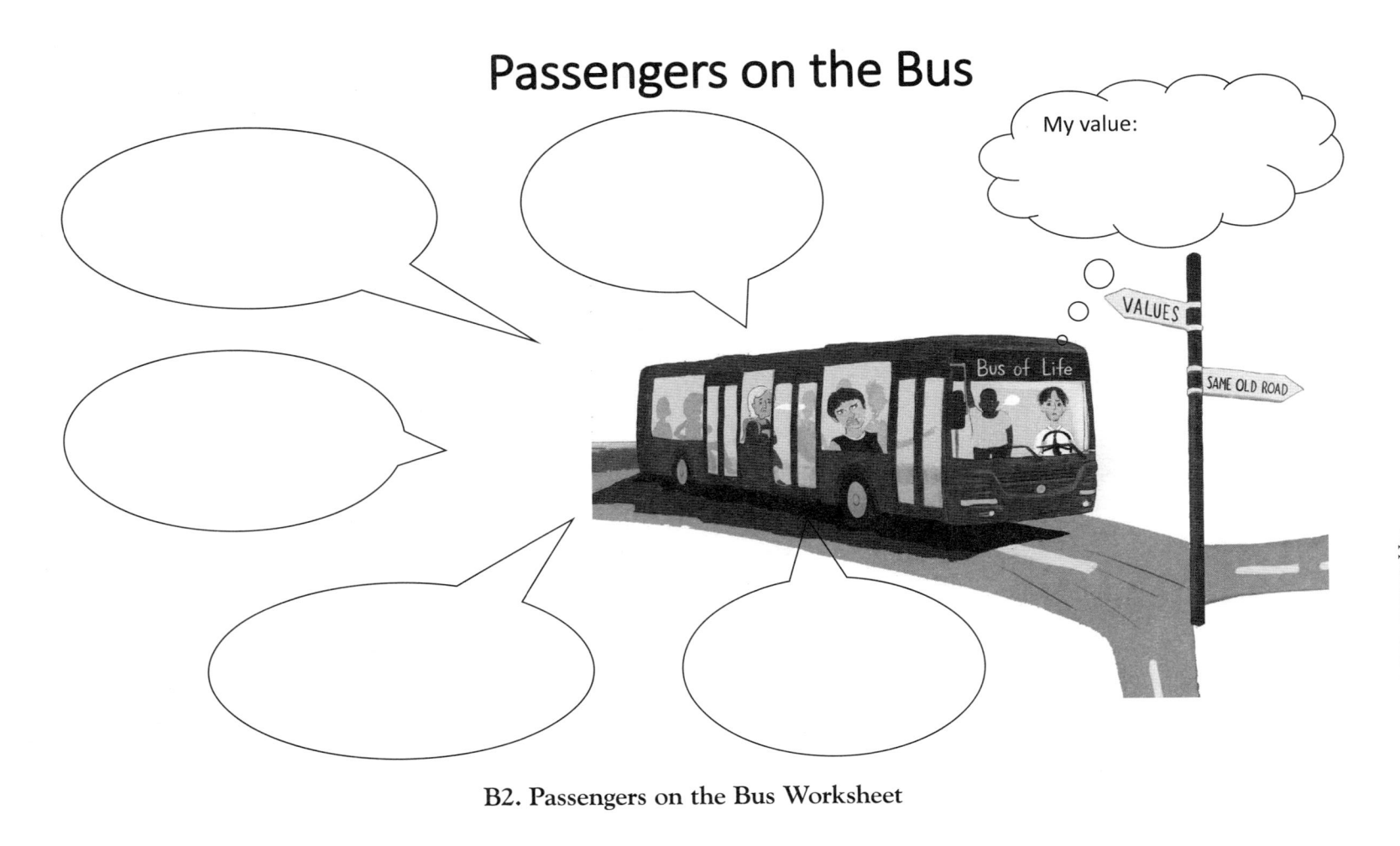

My value:

B2. Passengers on the Bus Worksheet

Committed Action Worksheet: Active

My SMART action for the week:
(specific, meaningful, adaptive, realistic, time-oriented)

Value(s) connected with my action:

Passengers that might come to the front of my bus:

B3. Committed Action Worksheet

Appendix B: Session Worksheets

Developing Aware Skills: Mindfulness Practice

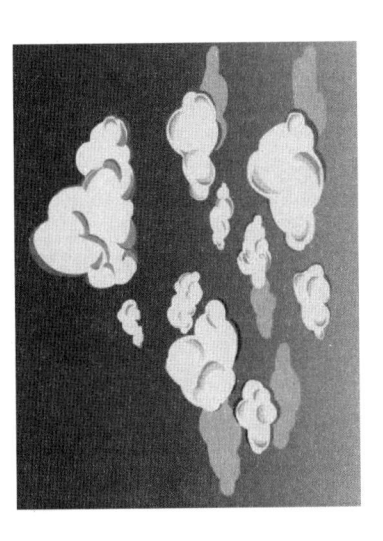

Mindfulness practice enables you to develop several skills:
- the ability to focus and engage in what you are doing
- the ability to let thoughts come and go without getting caught up in them
- the ability to refocus when you realize you're distracted
- the ability to let your feelings be as they are without trying to control them

The noticing exercise that I intend to practice this week:

You may find it helpful to record what you noticed during the mindfulness practice, and also any benefits you encounter that help you keep on track with getting active.

What I noticed (thoughts, feelings, sensations):

Benefits:

B4. Developing Aware Skills Worksheet

261

DRIVING LICENSE: Goals and Values

My life directions and goals:

_____
_____
_____

My actions to move me closer to my life goals:

_____
_____
_____

Values connected to my actions and life goals:

_____
_____
_____

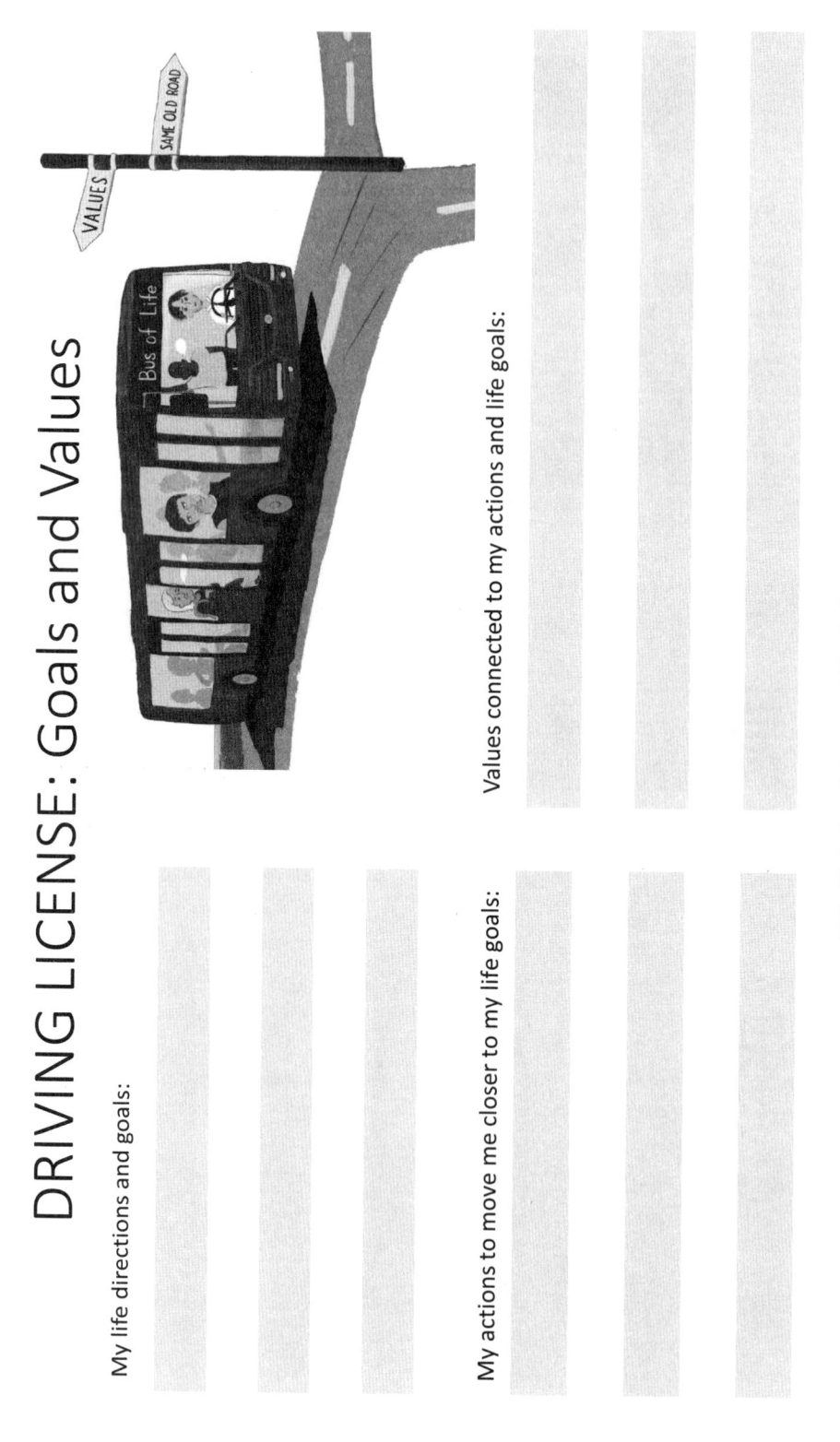

B5. Driving License Worksheet side 1

Appendix B: Session Worksheets

DRIVING LICENSE: Passengers

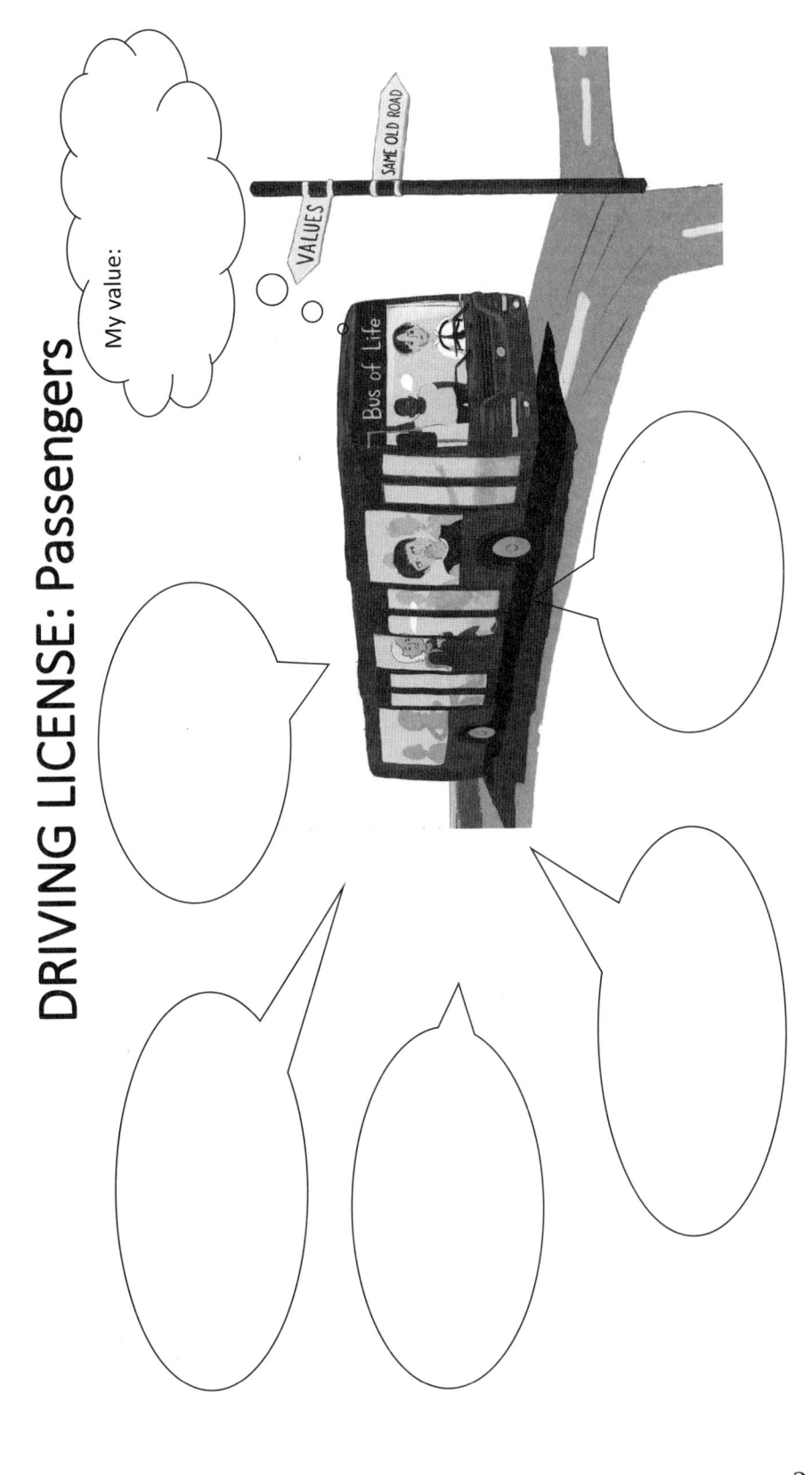

My value:

Bus of Life

VALUES / SAME OLD ROAD

B5. Driving License Worksheet side 2

263

Reference List

Abba, N., Chadwick, P., & Stevenson, C. (2008). Responding mindfully to distressing psychosis: A grounded theory analysis. *Psychotherapy Research, 18*, 77–87.

Albert, M., Becker, T., McCrone, P., & Thornicroft, G. (1998). Social networks and mental health service utilisation: A literature review. *International Journal of Social Psychiatry, 44*, 248–266.

Anthony, W. A. (1993). Recovery from mental illness: The guiding vision of the mental health service system in the 1990s. *Psychosocial Rehabilitation Journal, 16*, 11–23.

Askey, R., Holmshaw, J., Gamble, C., & Gray, R. (2009). What do carers of people with psychosis need from mental health services? Exploring the views of carers, service users and professionals. *Journal of Family Therapy, 31*, 310–331.

A-Tjak, J. G., Davis, M. L., Morina, N., Powers, M. B., Smits, J. A., & Emmelkamp P. M. (2015). A meta-analysis of the efficacy of acceptance and commitment therapy for clinically relevant mental and physical health problems. *Psychotherapy and Psychosomatics, 84*, 30–36.

Bach, P. A. (2004). ACT with the seriously mentally ill. In S. C. Hayes & K. D. Strosahl (Eds.), *A practical guide to acceptance and commitment therapy* (pp. 185–208). New York: Springer.

Bach, P., Gaudiano, B. A., Hayes, S. C., & Herbert, J. D. (2012). Acceptance and commitment therapy for psychosis: Intent to treat, hospitalization outcome and mediation by believability. *Psychosis, 5*, 166–174.

Bach, P., & Hayes, S. C. (2002). The use of acceptance and commitment therapy to prevent the rehospitalization of psychotic patients: A randomized controlled trial. *Journal of Consulting and Clinical Psychology, 70*, 1129–1139.

Bach, P., Hayes, S. C., & Gallop, R. (2012). Long-term effects of brief acceptance and commitment therapy for psychosis. *Behavior Modification, 36*, 165–181.

Bacon, T., Farhall, J., & Fossey, E. (2014). The active therapeutic processes of acceptance and commitment therapy for persistent symptoms of psychosis: Clients' perspectives. *Behavioural and Cognitive Psychotherapy, 42*, 402–420.

Baer, R. A., Smith, G. T., & Allen, K. B. (2004). Assessment of mindfulness by report: The Kentucky inventory of mindfulness skills. *Assessment, 11*, 191–206.

Barkham, M., Bewick, B., Mullin, T., Gilbody, S., Connell, J., Cahill, J., et al. (2013). The CORE–10: A short measure of psychological distress for routine use in the psychological therapies. *Counselling and Psychotherapy Research, 13*, 3–13.

Barton, K., & Jackson, C. (2008). Reducing symptoms of trauma among carers of people with psychosis: Pilot study examining the impact of writing about caregiving experiences. *Australian and New Zealand Journal of Psychiatry, 42*, 693–701.

Bates, A., Kemp, V., & Isaac, M. (2008). Peer support shows promise in helping persons living with mental illness address their physical health needs. *Canadian Journal of Community Mental Health, 27*, 21–36.

Bebbington, P., & Kuipers, L. (1994). The predictive utility of expressed emotion in schizophrenia: An aggregate analysis. *Psychological Medicine, 24*, 707–718.

Bentall, R. P. (2004). *Madness explained: Psychosis and human nature.* London: Penguin.

Berry, K., & Haddock, G. (2008). The implementation of the NICE guidelines for schizophrenia: Barriers to the implementation of psychological interventions and recommendations for the future. *Psychology and Psychotherapy: Theory, Research, and Practice, 81*, 419–436.

Birchwood, M. (2003). Pathways to emotional dysfunction in first-episode psychosis. *British Journal of Psychiatry, 182*, 373–375.

Birchwood, M., & Chadwick, P. (1997). The omnipotence of voices: Testing the validity of a cognitive model. *Psychological Medicine, 27*, 1345–1353.

Blackledge, J. T., Ciarrochi, J., & Deane, F. P. (2009). *Acceptance and commitment therapy: Contemporary theory, research and practice.* Bowen Hills: Australian Academic Press.

Blackledge, J. T., & Hayes, S. C. (2006). Using acceptance and commitment training in the support of parents of children diagnosed with autism. *Child and Family Behavior Therapy, 28*, 1–18.

Bond, F. W., Hayes, S. C., Baer, R. A., Carpenter, K. M., Guenole, N., Orcutt, H. K., et al. (2011). Preliminary psychometric properties of the Acceptance and Action Questionnaire-II: A revised measure of psychological inflexibility and experiential avoidance. *Behavior Therapy, 42*, 676–688.

Braham, L. G., Trower, P., & Birchwood, M. (2004). Acting on command hallucinations and dangerous behavior: A critique of the major findings in the last decade. *Clinical Psychology Review, 24*, 513–528.

Brassell, A. A., Rosenberg, E., Parent, J., Rough, J. N., Fondacaro, K., & Seehuus, M. (2016). Parent's psychological flexibility: Associations with parenting and child psychosocial well-being. *Journal of Contextual Behavioral Science, 5*, 111–120.

Brett, C. M. C., Peters, E. R., & McGuire P. K. (2015). Which psychotic experiences are associated with a need for clinical care? *European Psychiatry, 30*, 648–654.

British Psychological Society, Division of Clinical Psychology, & Cooke, A. (Ed.). (2014). *Understanding psychosis and schizophrenia: Why people sometimes hear voices, believe things that others find strange, or appear out of touch with reality, and what can help.* Leicester, UK: British Psychological Society.

Brown, K. W., & Ryan, R. M. (2003). The benefits of being present: Mindfulness and its role in psychological well-being. *Journal of Personality and Social Psychology, 84*, 822–848.

Brown, S., & Birtwistle, J. (1998). People with schizophrenia and their families: Fifteen-year outcome. *British Journal of Psychiatry, 173*, 139–144.

Butler, L., Johns, L. C., Byrne, M., Joseph, C., O'Donoghue, E., Jolley, S., et al. (2016). Running acceptance and commitment therapy groups for psychosis in community settings. *Journal of Contextual Behavioral Science, 5*, 33–38.

Butzlaff, R. L., & Hooley, J. M. (1998). Expressed emotion and psychiatric relapse: A meta-analysis. *Archives of General Psychiatry, 55*, 547–552.

Carers Trust. (2015). What is a carer? https://carers.org.

Cechnicki, A., Bielańska, A., Hanuszkiewicz, I., & Daren, A. (2013). The predictive validity of expressed emotions (EE) in schizophrenia: A 20-year prospective study. *Journal of Psychiatric Research, 47,* 208–214.

Chadwick, P. (2006). *Person-based cognitive therapy for distressing psychosis.* Chichester, UK: J. Wiley and Sons.

Chadwick, P., & Birchwood, M. (1994). The omnipotence of voices: A cognitive approach to auditory hallucinations. *British Journal of Psychiatry, 164,* 190–201.

Chadwick, P., & Birchwood, M. (1995). The omnipotence of voices II: The Beliefs About Voices Questionnaire (BAVQ). *British Journal of Psychiatry, 166,* 773–776.

Chadwick, P., Hember, M., Symes, J., Peters, E., Kuipers, E., & Dagnan, D. (2008). Responding mindfully to unpleasant thoughts and images: Reliability and validity of the Southampton Mindfulness Questionnaire (SMQ). *British Journal of Clinical Psychology, 47,* 451–455.

Chadwick, P., Newman-Taylor, K., & Abba, N. (2005). Mindfulness groups for people with psychosis. *Behavioural and Cognitive Psychotherapy, 33,* 351–359.

Chadwick, P., Strauss, C., Jones, A. M., Kingdon, D., Ellett, L., Dannahy, L., et al. (2016). Group mindfulness-based intervention for distressing voices: A pragmatic randomised controlled trial. *Schizophrenia Research, 175,* 168–173.

Clarke, S., Kingston, J., James, K., Bolderston, H., & Remington, B. (2014). Acceptance and commitment therapy group for treatment-resistant participants: A randomized controlled trial. *Journal of Contextual Behavioral Science, 3,* 179–188.

Cohen, C. I., & Berk, L. A. (1985). Personal coping styles of schizophrenic outpatients. *Hospital and Community Psychiatry, 36,* 407–410.

Corstens, D., Longden, E., & May, R. (2012). Talking with voices: Exploring what is expressed by the voices people hear. *Psychosis: Psychological, Social and Integrative Approaches, 4,* 95–104.

Cramer, H., Lauche, R., Haller, H., Langhorst, J., & Dobos, G. (2016). Mindfulness- and acceptance-based interventions for psychosis: A systematic review and meta-analysis. *Global Advances in Health and Medicine, 5,* 30–43.

Crawford, P., Gilbert, P., Gilbert, J., Gale, C., & Harvey, K. (2016). The language of compassion in acute mental health care. *Qualitative Health Research, 23,* 719–727.

Crepaz Keay, D., & Cyhlarova, E. (2012). A new self-management intervention for people with severe psychiatric diagnoses. *Journal of Mental Health Training, Education and Practice, 7,* 89–94.

Csipke, E., Flach, C., McCrone, P., Rose, D., Tilley, J., Wykes, T., et al. (2014). Inpatient care 50 years after the process of deinstitutionalisation. *Social Psychiatry and Psychiatric Epidemiology, 49,* 665–671.

Dannahy, L., Hayward, M., Strauss, C., Turton, W., Harding, E., & Chadwick, P. (2011). Group person-based cognitive therapy for distressing voices: Pilot data from nine groups. *Journal of Behavior Therapy and Experimental Psychiatry, 42,* 111–116.

Davidson, L., Bellamy, C., Guy, K., & Miller, R. (2012). Peer support among persons with severe mental illnesses: A review of evidence and experience. *World Psychiatry, 11,* 123–128.

Deegan, P. E. (1988). Recovery: The lived experience of rehabilitation. *Psychosocial Rehabilitation Journal, 11*, 11–19.

Dimsdale, J. E., Klerman, G., & Shershow, J. G. (1979). Conflict in treatment goals between patients and staff. *Social Psychiatry, 14*, 1–4.

Dixon, L. B., Dickerson, F., Bellack, A. S., Bennett, M., Dickinson, D., Goldberg, R. W., et al. (2010). The 2009 schizophrenia PORT psychosocial treatment recommendations and summary statements. *Schizophrenia Bulletin, 36*, 48–70.

Dudley, D., Taylor, P., Wickham, S., & Hutton, P. (2015). Psychosis, delusions and the "jumping to conclusions" reasoning bias: A systematic review and meta-analysis. *Schizophrenia Bulletin, 42*, 652–665.

Escher, S., Delespaul, P., Romme, M., Buiks, A., & van Os, J. (2003). Coping defence and depression in adolescents hearing voices. *Journal of Mental Health, 12*, 91–99.

Farhall, J., & Gehrke, M. (1997). Coping with hallucinations: Exploring stress and coping framework. *British Journal of Clinical Psychology, 36*, 259–261.

Farhall, J., Shawyer, F., Thomas, N., & Morris, E. M. J. (2013). Clinical assessment and assessment measures. In E. M. J. Morris, L. C. Johns, & J. E. Oliver (Eds.), *Acceptance and commitment therapy and mindfulness for psychosis* (pp. 47–63). Chichester, UK: Wiley-Blackwell.

Faulkner, A., & Basset, T. (2012). A long and honourable history. *Journal of Mental Health Education and Training, 7*, 53–59.

Fletcher, L., & Hayes, S. C. (2005). Relational frame theory, acceptance and commitment therapy, and a functional analytic definition of mindfulness. *Journal of Rational-Emotive and Cognitive-Behavior Therapy, 23*, 315–336.

Forchuk, C., Reynolds, W., Sharkey, S., Martin, M., & Jensen, E. (2007). Transitional discharge based on therapeutic relationships: State of the art. *Archives of Psychiatric Nursing, 21*, 80–86.

Frederick, J., & Cotanch, P. (1995). Self-help strategies for auditory hallucinations in schizophrenia. *Issues in Mental Health Nursing, 16*, 213–224.

Freeman, D., Dunn, G., Startup, H., Pugh, K., Cordwell, J., Mander, H., et al. (2015). Effects of cognitive behaviour therapy for worry on persecutory delusions in patients with psychosis (WIT): a parallel, single-blind, randomised controlled trial with a mediation analysis. *Lancet Psychiatry, 2*, 305–313.

Freeman, D., Garety, P. A., Fowler, D., Kuipers, E., Bebbington, P. E., & Dunn, G. (2004). Why do people with delusions fail to choose more realistic explanations for their experiences? An empirical investigation. *Journal of Consulting and Clinical Psychology, 72*, 671–680.

Furukawa, T. A., Levine, S. Z., Tanaka, S., Goldberg, Y., Samara, M., Davis, J. M., et al. (2015). Initial severity of schizophrenia and efficacy of antipsychotics: Participant-level meta-analysis of 6 placebo-controlled studies. *JAMA Psychiatry, 72*, 14–21.

Gaebel, W., Riesbeck, M., & Wobrock, T. (2011). Schizophrenia guidelines across the world: A selective review and comparison. *International Review of Psychiatry, 23*, 379–387.

Galletly, C., Castle, D., Dark, F., Humberstone, V., Jablensky, A., Killackey, E., et al. (2016). Royal Australian and New Zealand College of Psychiatrists clinical practice guidelines for the management of schizophrenia and related disorders. *Australian and New Zealand Journal of Psychiatry, 50*, 410–472.

García-Montes, J. M., Luciano Soriano, M. C., Hernández-López, M., & Zaldívar, F. (2004). Aplicación de la terapia de aceptación y compromiso (ACT) a sintomatología delirante: Un estudio de caso [Application of acceptance and commitment therapy (ACT) in delusional symptomathology: A case study]. *Psicothema, 16*, 117–124.

García-Montes, J. M., Pérez-Álvarez, M., & Perona-Garcelán, S. (2013). Acceptance and commitment therapy for delusions. In E. Morris, L. Johns, & J. Oliver (Eds.), *Acceptance and commitment therapy and mindfulness for psychosis*. Chichester, UK: Wiley-Blackwell.

Garety, P. A., Fowler, D. G., Freeman, D., Bebbington, P., Dunn, G., & Kuipers, E. (2008). Cognitive-behavioural therapy and family intervention for relapse prevention and symptom reduction in psychosis: Randomised controlled trial. *British Journal of Psychiatry, 192*, 412–423.

Garety, P., Fowler, D., & Kuipers, E. (2000). Cognitive-behavioral therapy for medication-resistant symptoms. *Schizophrenia Bulletin, 26*, 73–86.

Gaudiano, B. A., & Herbert, J. D. (2006). Acute treatment of inpatients with psychotic symptoms using acceptance and commitment therapy: Pilot results. *Behaviour Research and Therapy, 44*, 415–437.

Gaudiano, B. A., Herbert, J. D., & Hayes, S. C. (2010). Is it the symptom or the relation to it? Investigating potential mediators of change in acceptance and commitment therapy for psychosis. *Behavior Therapy, 41*, 543–554.

Gilbert, H. (2015). *Mental health under pressure*. London: King's Fund.

Gilbert, P., Birchwood, M., Gilbert, J., Trower, P., Hay, J., Murray, B., et al. (2001). An exploration of evolved mental mechanisms for dominant and subordinate behaviour in relation to auditory hallucinations in schizophrenia and critical thoughts in depression. *Psychological Medicine, 31*, 1117–1127.

Gillanders, D. T., Bolderston, H., Bond, F. W., Dempster, M., Flaxman, P. E., Campbell, L., et al. (2014). The development and initial validation of the Cognitive Fusion Questionnaire. *Behavior Therapy, 45*, 83–101.

Giron, M., Fernandez-Yanez, A., Mana-Alvarenga, S., Molina-Habas, A., Nolasco, A., & Gomez-Beneyto, M. (2010). Efficacy and effectiveness of individual family intervention on social and clinical functioning and family burden in severe schizophrenia: A 2-year randomized controlled study. *Psychological Medicine, 40*, 73–84.

Glynn, S. M. (2012). Family interventions in schizophrenia: Promise and pitfalls over 30 years. *Current Psychiatry Reports, 14*, 237–243.

Goldsmith, L. P., Lewis, S. W., Dunn, G., & Bentall, R. P. (2015). Psychological treatments for early psychosis can be beneficial or harmful, depending on the therapeutic alliance: An instrumental variable analysis. *Psychological Medicine, 45*, 2365–2673.

Great Britain Department of Health. (2006). *Reward and recognition: The principles and practice of service user payment and reimbursement in health and social care, a guide for service providers, service users and carers*. London: Great Britain, Department of Health.

Gumley, A., White, R., Briggs, A., Ford, I., Barry, S., Stewart, C., et al. (2016). A parallel group randomised open blinded evaluation of acceptance and commitment therapy for depression after psychosis: A pilot trial protocol (ADAPT). *Psychosis, 8*, 143–155.

Hacker, D., Birchwood, M., Tudway, J., Meaden, A., & Amphlett, C. (2008). Acting on voices: Omnipotence, sources of threat, and safety-seeking behaviours. *British Journal of Clinical Psychology, 47,* 201–213.

Haddock, G., Slade, P. D., Bentall, R. P., Reid, D., & Faragher, E. B. (1998). A comparison of the long-term effectiveness of distraction and focusing in the treatment of auditory hallucinations. *British Journal of Medical Psychology, 71,* 339–349.

Harris, R. (2014). The happiness trap: Values, goals and barriers cards. https://www.actmindfully.com.au/bookshop_detail.asp?id=1100&catid=97.

Hayes, S. C. (2004). Acceptance and commitment therapy, relational frame theory, and the third wave of behavioral and cognitive therapies. *Behavior Therapy, 35,* 639–665.

Hayes, S. C., Luoma, J. B., Bond, F. W., Masuda, A., & Lillis, J. (2006). Acceptance and commitment therapy: Model, processes and outcomes. *Behaviour Research and Therapy, 44,* 1–25.

Hayes, S. C., & Shenk, C. (2004). Operationalizing mindfulness without unnecessary attachments. *Clinical Psychology: Science and Practice, 11,* 249–254.

Hayes, S. C., Strosahl, K., & Wilson, K. G. (1999). *Acceptance and commitment therapy: An experiential approach to behavior change.* New York: Guilford Press.

Hayes, S. C., Strosahl, K., & Wilson, K. G. (2012). *Acceptance and commitment therapy: The process and practice of mindful change.* New York: Guilford Press.

Hayes, S. C., Villatte, M., Levin, M., & Hildebrandt, M. (2011). Open, aware and active: Contextual approaches as an emerging trend in the behavioral and cognitive therapies. *Annual Review of Clinical Psychology, 7,* 141–168.

Hileman, J. W., Lackey, N. R., & Hassanein, R. S. (1992). Identifying the needs of home caregivers of patients with cancer. *Oncology Nursing Forum, 19,* 771–777.

Hjorthøj, C., Stürup, A. E., McGrath, J. J., & Nordentoft, M. (2017). Years of potential life lost and life expectancy in schizophrenia: A systematic review and meta-analysis. *Lancet Psychiatry, 4,* 295–301.

Hsiao, C. Y., & Tsai, Y. F. (2014). Caregiver burden and satisfaction in families of individuals with schizophrenia. *Nursing Research, 63,* 260–269.

Ince, P., Haddock, G., & Tai, S. (2015). A systematic review of the implementation of recommended psychological interventions for schizophrenia: Rates, barriers, and improvement strategies. *Psychology and Psychotherapy: Theory, Research and Practice, 89,* 324–350.

Ingham, B., Riley, J., Nevin, H., Evans, G., & Gair, E. (2013). An initial evaluation of direct care staff resilience workshops in intellectual disabilities services. *Journal of Intellectual Disabilities, 17,* 214–222.

Jääskeläinen, A. E., Juola, P., Hirvonen, N., McGrath, J. J., Saha, S., Isohanni, M., et al. (2013). Systematic review and meta-analysis of recovery in schizophrenia. *Schizophrenia Bulletin, 39,* 1296–1306.

Jacobsen, P., Morris, E., Johns, L., & Hodkinson, K. (2011). Mindfulness groups for psychosis; key issues for implementation on an inpatient unit. *Behavioural and Cognitive Psychotherapy, 39,* 349–353.

Jauhar, S., McKenna, P. J., Radua, J., Fung, E., Salvador, R., & Laws, K. R. (2014). Cognitive-behavioural therapy for the symptoms of schizophrenia: Systematic review and meta-analysis with examination of potential bias. *British Journal of Psychiatry, 204,* 20–29.

Johns, L. C., Jolley, S., Keen, N., & Peters, E. (2014). CBT with people with psychosis. In A. Whittington & N. Grey (Eds.), *How to become a more effective CBT therapist: Mastering metacompetence in clinical practice* (pp. 191–207). Chichester, UK: Wiley-Blackwell.

Johns, L. C., Oliver, J. E., Khondoker, M., Byrne, M., Jolley, S., Wykes, T., et al. (2015). The feasibility and acceptability of a brief acceptance and commitment therapy (ACT) group intervention for people with psychosis: The "ACT for Life" study. *Journal of Behavior Therapy and Experimental Psychiatry, 50,* 257–263.

Jolley, S., Garety, P. A., Ellett, L., Kuipers, E., Freeman, D., Bebbington, P. E., et al. (2006). A validation of a new measure of activity in psychosis. *Schizophrenia Research, 85,* 288–295.

Jolley, S., Garety, P., Peters, E., Fornells-Ambrojo, M., Onwumere, J., Harris, V., et al. (2015). Opportunities and challenges in Improving Access to Psychological Therapies for people with Severe Mental Illness (IAPT-SMI): Evaluating the first operational year of the South London and Maudsley (SLaM) demonstration site for psychosis. *Behaviour Research and Therapy, 64,* 24–30.

Jolley, S., Johns, L. C., O'Donoghue, E., Oliver, J., Khondoker, M., Byrne, M., et al. (in press). Acceptance and commitment therapy for patients and caregivers in psychosis services: A randomised controlled trial. *Journal of Behavior Therapy and Experimental Psychiatry.*

Jolley, S., Onwumere, J., Bissoli, S., Bhayani, P., Singh, G., Kuipers, E., et al. (2015). A pilot evaluation of therapist training in cognitive therapy for psychosis: Therapy quality and clinical outcomes. *Behavioural and Cognitive Psychotherapy, 43,* 478–489.

Kabat-Zinn, J. (1994). *Wherever you go, there you are: Mindfulness meditation in everyday life.* New York: Hyperion.

Kabat-Zinn, J. (2003). Mindfulness–based interventions in context: Past, present, and future. *Clinical Psychology Science and Practice, 10,* 144–156.

Kashdan, T. B., & Rottenberg, J. (2010). Psychological flexibility as a fundamental aspect of health. *Clinical Psychology Review, 30,* 865–878.

Kelleher, I., & DeVylder, J. E. (2017). Hallucinations in borderline personality disorder and common mental disorders. *British Journal of Psychiatry, 210,* 230–231.

Khoury, B., Lecomte, T., Fortin, G., Masse, M., Therien, P., Bouchard, V., et al. (2013). Mindfulness-based therapy: A comprehensive meta-analysis. *Clinical Psychology Review, 33,* 763–771.

Kingdon, D. G., & Turkington, D. (1994). *Cognitive-behavioral therapy of schizophrenia.* New York: Guilford Press.

Knapp, M., Andrew, A., McDaid, D., Iemmi, V., McCrone, P., Park, A-La, et al. (2014). *Investing in recovery: Making the business case for effective interventions for people with schizophrenia and psychosis.* London: PSSRU, The London School of Economics and Political Science, and Centre for Mental Health.

Kroeker, G. (2009). Reservoir metaphor. *Garth Kroeker* (blog), January 25. http://garthkroeker.blogspot.co.uk/2009_01_01_archive.html.

Kuipers, E., Onwumere, J., & Bebbington, P. (2010). Cognitive model of caregiving in psychosis. *British Journal of Psychiatry, 196,* 259–265.

Kulhara, P., Chakrabarti, S., Avasthi, A., Sharma, A., & Sharma, S. (2009). Psychoeducational intervention for caregivers of Indian patients with schizophrenia: A randomised–controlled trial. *Acta Psychiatrica Scandinavica, 119,* 472–483.

Laidlaw, T. M., Coverdale, J. H., Falloon, I. R., & Kydd, R. R. (2002). Caregivers' stresses when living together or apart from patients with chronic schizophrenia. *Community Mental Health Journal, 38*, 303–310.

Lamb, H. R., & Bachrach, L. L. (2001). Some perspectives on deinstitutionalization. *Psychiatric Services, 52*, 1039–1045.

Larsen, D. L., Attkisson, C. C., Hargreaves, W. A., & Nguyen, T. D. (1979). Assessment of client/patient satisfaction: Development of a general scale. *Evaluation and Program Planning, 2*, 197–207.

Lauber, C., Eichenberger, A., Luginbühl, P., Keller, C., & Rössler, W. (2003). Determinants of burden in caregivers of patients with exacerbating schizophrenia. *European Psychiatry, 18*, 285–289.

Lavis, A. (2015). Careful starving: Reflections on (not) eating, caring and anorexia. In E.-J. Abbots, A. Lavis, & L. Attala (Eds.), *Careful eating: Bodies, food and care* (pp. 91–108). Surrey, UK: Ashgate.

Lawn, S., Smith, A., & Hunter, K. (2008). Mental health peer support for hospital avoidance and early discharge: An Australian example of consumer driven and operated service. *Journal of Mental Health, 17*, 498–508.

Leamy, M., Bird, V., Le Boutillier, C., Williams, J., & Slade, M. (2011). Conceptual framework for personal recovery in mental health: Systematic review and narrative synthesis. *British Journal of Psychiatry, 199*, 445–452.

Lee, G., Barrowclough, C., & Lobban, F. (2014). Positive affect in the family environment protects against relapse in first-episode psychosis. *Social Psychiatry and Psychiatric Epidemiology, 49*, 367–376.

Lester, P., Leskin, G., Woodward, K., Saltzman, W., Nash, W., Mogil, C., et al. (2011). Wartime deployment and military children: Applying prevention science to enhance family resilience. In S. M. Wadsworth & D. Riggs (Eds.), *Risk and resilience in US military families* (pp. 149–173). New York: Springer.

Levin, M. E., Hildebrandt, M. J., Lillis, J., & Hayes, S. C. (2012). The impact of treatment components suggested by the psychological flexibility model: A meta-analysis of laboratory-based component studies. *Behavior Therapy, 43*, 741–756.

Lieberman, J. A., Stroup, T. S., McEvoy, J. P., Swartz, M. S., Rosenheck, R. A., Perkins, D. O., et al. (2005). Effectiveness of antipsychotic drugs in patients with chronic schizophrenia. *New England Journal of Medicine, 353*, 1209–1223.

Linehan, M. (1993). *Cognitive-behavioral treatment of borderline personality disorder.* New York: Guilford Press.

Linscott, R. J., & van Os, J. (2013). An updated and conservative systematic review and meta-analysis of epidemiological evidence on psychotic experiences in children and adults: On the pathway from proneness to persistence to dimensional expression across mental disorders. *Psychological Medicine, 1*, 1–17.

Longden, E., Corstens, D., Escher, S., & Romme, M. (2012). Voice hearing in biographical context: A model for formulating the relationship between voices and life history. *Psychosis: Psychological, Social and Integrative Approaches, 4*, 224–234.

Losada, A., Márquez-González, M., Romero-Moreno, R., Mausbach, B. T., López, J., Fernández-Fernández, V., et al. (2015). Cognitive-behavioral therapy (CBT) versus acceptance and commitment therapy (ACT) for dementia family caregivers with significant depressive symptoms: Results of a randomized clinical trial. *Journal of Consulting and Clinical Psychology, 83*, 760–772.

Luoma, J. B., Hayes, S. C., & Walser, R. D. (2007). *Learning ACT: An acceptance and commitment therapy skills-training manual for therapists.* Oakland, CA: Context Press.

Martin, J. A., & Penn, D. L. (2002). Attributional style in schizophrenia: An investigation in outpatients with and without persecutory delusions. *Schizophrenia Bulletin, 28*, 131–141.

McAndrew, S., Chambers, M., Nolan, F., Thomas, B., & Watts, P. (2014). Measuring the evidence: Reviewing the literature of the measurement of therapeutic engagement in acute mental health inpatient wards. *International Journal of Mental Health Nursing, 23*, 212–220.

McArthur, A., Mitchell, G., & Johns, L. C. (2013). Developing acceptance and commitment therapy for psychosis as a group-based intervention. In E. M. J. Morris., L. C. Johns., & J. E. Oliver (Eds.), *Acceptance and commitment therapy and mindfulness for psychosis* (pp. 219–239). Chichester, UK: Wiley-Blackwell.

McCrone, P., Craig, T. K., Power, P., & Garety, P. A. (2010). Cost-effectiveness of an early intervention service for people with psychosis. *British Journal of Psychiatry, 196*, 377–382.

McGrath, J. J., Saha, S., Al-Hamzawi, A., Alonso, J., Bromet, E. J., Bruffaerts, R., et al. (2015). Psychotic experiences in the general population: A cross-national analysis based on 31,261 respondents from 18 countries. *JAMA Psychiatry, 72*, 697–705.

Merwin, R. M., Zucker, N. L., & Timko, C. A. (2013). A pilot study of an acceptance-based separated family treatment for adolescent anorexia nervosa. *Cognitive and Behavioral Practice, 20*, 485–500.

Mistry, H., Levack, W. M. M., & Johnson, S. (2015). Enabling people, not completing tasks: Patient perspectives on relationships and staff morale in mental health wards in England. *BMC Psychiatry, 15*, 307–316.

Mitchell, G., & McArthur, A. (2013). Acceptance and commitment therapy for psychosis in acute psychiatric admission settings. In E. M. J. Morris, L. C. Johns, & J. E. Oliver (Eds.), *Acceptance and commitment therapy and mindfulness for psychosis* (pp. 206–218). Chichester, UK: Wiley-Blackwell.

Morgan, C., Lappin, J., Heslin, M., Donoghue, K., Lomas, B., Reininghaus, U., et al. (2014). Reappraising the long-term course and outcome of psychotic disorders: The AESOP-10 study. *Psychological Medicine, 44*, 2713–2726.

Morris, E. M. J., & Bilich-Eric, L. (2017). A framework to support experiential learning and psychological flexibility in supervision: SHAPE. *Australian Psychologist, 52*, 104–113.

Morris, E. M. J., Garety, P., & Peters, E. (2014). Psychological flexibility and non-judgemental acceptance in voice-hearers: Relationships with omnipotence and distress. *Australian and New Zealand Journal of Psychiatry, 48*, 1150–1156.

Morris, E. M. J., Johns, L. C., & Oliver, J. E. (Eds.). (2013). *Acceptance and commitment therapy and mindfulness for psychosis.* Chichester, UK: John Wiley and Sons.

Morrison, A. P., & Haddock, G. (1997). Cognitive factors in source monitoring and auditory hallucinations. *Psychological Medicine, 27*, 669–679.

National Institute for Health and Care Excellence (2014). *Psychosis and schizophrenia in adults: Treatment and management (CG178)*. London: National Institute for Health and Care Excellence.

Nayani, T., & David, A. S. (1996). The auditory hallucination: A phenomenological survey. *Psychological Medicine, 26*, 177–189.

Neil, S. T., Kilbride, M., Pitt, L., Nothard, S., Welford, M., Sellwood, W., et al. (2009). The Questionnaire about the Process of Recovery (QPR): A measurement tool developed in collaboration with service users. *Psychosis, 1*, 145–155.

Newell, S. E., Harries, P., & Ayers, S. (2012). Boredom proneness in a psychiatric inpatient population. *International Journal of Social Psychiatry, 58*, 488–495.

NHS England. (2013). Introduction to the Friends and Family Test. https://www.england.nhs.uk/ourwork/pe/fft.

Noone, S. J., & Hastings, R. P. (2010). Using acceptance and mindfulness-based workshops with support staff caring for adults with intellectual disabilities. *Mindfulness, 1*, 67–73.

Nordentoft, M., Madsen, T., & Fedyszyn, I. (2015). Suicidal behavior and mortality in first-episode psychosis. *Journal of Nervous and Mental Disease, 203*, 387–392.

Norman, R. M., Malla, A. K., Manchanda, R., Harricharan, R., Takhar, J., & Northcott, S. (2005). Social support and three-year symptom and admission outcomes for first episode psychosis. *Schizophrenia Research, 80*, 227–234.

Novella, E. J. (2010). Mental health care and the politics of inclusion: A social systems account of psychiatric deinstitutionalization. *Theoretical Medicine and Bioethics, 31*, 411–427.

Oliver, J. E., Hayward, M., McGuiness, H. B., & Strauss, C. (2013). The service user experience of acceptance and commitment therapy and person-based cognitive therapy. In E. M. J. Morris., L. C. Johns, & J. E. Oliver (Eds.), *Acceptance and commitment therapy and mindfulness for psychosis* (pp. 172–189). Chichester, UK: Wiley-Blackwell.

Oliver, J. E., O'Connor, J. A., Jose, P. E., McLachlan, K., & Peters, E. R. (2012). The impact of negative schemas, mood and psychological flexibility on delusional ideation: Mediating and moderating effects. *Psychosis, 4*, 6–18.

Oliver, J. E., Venter, J. H., & Lloyd, L. (2014). An evaluation of a training workshop for delivering group-based interventions for NHS staff. *Clinical Psychology Forum, 257*, 40–44.

Onwumere, J., Grice, S., & Kuipers, E. (2016). Delivering cognitive–behavioural family interventions for schizophrenia. *Australian Psychologist, 51*, 52–61.

Onwumere, J., Lotey, G., Schulz, J., James, G., Afsharzadegan, R., Harvey, R., et al. (2015). Burnout in early course psychosis caregivers: The role of illness beliefs and coping styles. *Early Intervention in Psychiatry*, DOI: 10.1111/eip.12227.

Onwumere, J., Shiers, D., & Chew-Graham, C. (2016). Understanding the needs of carers of people with psychosis in primary care. *British Journal of General Practice, 66*, 400–401.

Ost, L. G. (2014). The efficacy of acceptance and commitment therapy: An updated systematic review and meta-analysis. *Behaviour Research and Therapy, 61*, 105–121.

Owen, M., Sellwood, W., Kan, S., Murray, J., & Sarsam, M. (2015). Group CBT for psychosis: A longitudinal, controlled trial with inpatients. *Behaviour Research and Therapy, 65*, 76–85.

Pankey, J., & Hayes, S. (2003). Acceptance and commitment therapy for psychosis. *International Journal of Psychology and Psychological Therapy, 3*, 311–328.

Patterson, P., Birchwood, M., & Cochrane, R. (2005). Expressed emotion as an adaptation to loss. *British Journal of Psychiatry, 187*, s59–s64.

Pérez-Álvarez, M., García-Montes, J. M., Perona-Garcelán, S., & Vallina-Fernández, O. (2008). Changing relationship with voices: New therapeutic perspectives for treating hallucinations. *Clinical Psychology and Psychotherapy, 15*, 75–85.

Perkins, R. (2001). What constitutes success? The relative priority of service users' and clinicians' views of mental health services. *British Journal of Psychiatry, 179*, 9–10.

Pharoah, F., Mari, J., Rathbone, J., & Wong, W. (2010). Family intervention for schizophrenia. *Cochrane Database of Systematic Reviews, 12*, CD000088.

Poon, A. W., Harvey, C., Mackinnon, A., & Joubert, L. (2016). A longitudinal population-based study of carers of people with psychosis. *Epidemiology and Psychiatric Sciences*, DOI: 10.1017/S2045796015001195.

Price, L. M. (2007). Transition to community: A program to help clients with schizophrenia move from inpatient to community care; a pilot study. *Archives of Psychiatric Nursing, 21*, 336–344.

Priebe, S., Huxley, P., Knight, S., & Evans, S. (1999). Application and results of the Manchester Short Assessment of Quality of Life (MANSA). *International Journal of Social Psychiatry, 45*, 7–12.

Prytys, M., Garety, P. A., Jolley, S., Onwumere, J., & Craig, T. (2011). Implementing the NICE guideline for schizophrenia recommendations for psychological therapies: A qualitative analysis of the attitudes of CMHT staff. *Clinical Psychology and Psychotherapy, 18*, 48–59.

Radcliffe, J., & Smith, R. (2007). Acute in-patient psychiatry: How patients spend their time on acute psychiatric wards. *Psychiatric Bulletin, 31*, 167–170.

Reynolds, W., Lauder, W., Sharkey, S., Maciver, S., Veitch, T., & Cameron, D. (2004). The effects of a transitional discharge model for psychiatric patients. *Journal of Psychiatric and Mental Health Nursing, 11*, 82–88.

Romme, M., & Escher, A. (1989). Hearing voices. *Schizophrenia Bulletin, 15*, 209–216.

Romme, M., & Escher, S. (1993). *Accepting voices*. London: Mind Publications.

Romme, M., Honig, A., Noorthoorn, E. O., & Escher, A. D. (1992). Coping with hearing voices: An emancipatory approach. *British Journal of Psychiatry, 161*, 99–103.

Rosen, A. (2006). The Australian experience of the deinstitutionalization: Interaction of Australian culture with the development and reform of its mental health services. *Acta Psychiatrica Scandinavica, 113*, 81–89.

Ruddle, A., Mason, O., & Wykes, T. (2011). A review of hearing voices groups: Evidence and mechanisms of change. *Clinical Psychology Review, 31*, 757–766.

Schene, A. H., van Wijngaarden, B., & Koeter, M. W. (1998). Family caregiving in schizophrenia: Domains and distress. *Schizophrenia Bulletin, 24*, 609–618.

Schizophrenia Commission. (2012). *The abandoned illness: A report from the Schizophrenia Commission*. London: Rethink Mental Illness.

Schofield, N., Quinn, J., Haddock, G., & Barrowclough, C. (2001). Schizophrenia and substance misuse problems: A comparison between patients with and without significant carer contact. *Social Psychiatry and Psychiatric Epidemiology, 36*, 523–528.

Sealy, P., & Whitehead, P. C. (2004). Forty years of deinstitutionalization of psychiatric services in Canada: An empirical assessment. *Canadian Journal of Psychiatry, 49*, 249–257.

Segal, Z. V., Williams, J. M. G., & Teasdale, J. D. (2002). *Mindfulness-based cognitive therapy for depression.* New York: Guildford Press.

Shawyer, F., Farhall, J., Mackinnon, A., Trauer, T., Sims, E., Ratcliff, K., et al. (2012). A randomised controlled trial of acceptance-based cognitive behavioural therapy for command hallucinations in psychotic disorders. *Behaviour Research and Therapy, 50*, 110–121.

Shawyer, F., Farhall, J., Thomas, N., Hayes, S. C., Gallop, R., Copolov, D., et al. (2017). Acceptance and commitment therapy for psychosis: Randomised controlled trial. *British Journal of Psychiatry, 210*, 140–148.

Shawyer, F., Mackinnon, A., Farhall, J., Sims, E., Blaney, S., Yardley, P., et al. (2008). Acting on harmful command hallucinations in psychotic disorders: An integrative approach. *Journal of Nervous and Mental Disease, 196*, 390–398.

Sheehan, D. V. (1983). *The anxiety disease.* New York: Charles Scribner and Sons.

Sheehan, D. V., Harnett-Sheehan, K., & Raj, B. A. (1996). The measurement of disability. *International Clinical Psychopharmacology, 11*, 89–95.

Sheehan, K. H., & Sheehan, D. V. (2008). Assessing treatment effects in clinical trials with the discan metric of the Sheehan Disability Scale. *International Clinical Psychopharmacology, 23*, 70–83.

Simpson, E. L., & House, A. O. (2002). Involving users in the delivery and evaluation of mental health services: Systematic review. *British Medical Journal, 325*, 1265–1267.

Sin, J., & Norman, I. (2013). Psychoeducational interventions for family members of people with schizophrenia: A mixed-method systematic review. *Journal of Clinical Psychiatry, 74*, 1145–1162.

Slade, M. (2009). *Personal recovery and mental illness: A guide for mental health professionals.* Cambridge: Cambridge University Press.

Smout, M., Davies, M., Burns, N., & Christie, A. (2014). Development of the Valuing Questionnaire (VQ). *Journal of Contextual Behavioral Science, 3*, 164–172.

Stewart-Brown, S. L., Platt, S., Tennant, A., Maheswaran, H., Parkinson, J., Weich, S., et al. (2011). The Warwick-Edinburgh Mental Well-Being Scale (WEMWBS): A valid and reliable tool for measuring mental well-being in diverse populations and projects. *Journal of Epidemiology and Community Health, 65*, A38–A39.

Strauss, C., Thomas, N., & Hayward, M. (2015). Can we respond mindfully to distressing voices? A systematic review of evidence for engagement, acceptability, effectiveness and mechanisms of change for mindfulness-based interventions for people distressed by hearing voices. *Frontiers in Psychology, 6*, Article 1154.

Tait, L., & Lester, H. (2005). Encouraging user involvement in mental health services. *Advances in Psychiatric Treatment, 11*, 168–175.

Taylor Salisbury, T., Killaspy, H., & King, M. (2016). An international comparison of the deinstitutionalisation of mental health care: Development and findings of the Mental

Health Services Denationalisation Measure (MENDit). *BMC Psychiatry, 16*, DOI: 10.1186/s12888-016-0762-4.

Teasdale, J. D. (1999). Emotional processing, three modes of mind and the prevention of relapse in depression. *Behaviour Research and Therapy, 37*, S53–S77.

Tennant, R., Hiller, L., Fishwick, R., Platt, S., Joseph, S., Weich, S., et al. (2007). The Warwick-Edinburgh Mental Well-Being Scale (WEMWBS): Development and UK validation. *Health and Quality of Life Outcomes, 5*, DOI: 10.1186/1477-7525-5-63.

Theodore, K., Johnson, S., Chalmers-Brown, A., Doherty, R., Harrop, C., & Ellett, L. (2012). Quality of life and illness beliefs in individuals with early psychosis. *Social Psychiatry and Psychiatric Epidemiology, 47*, 545–551.

Thomas, N., Morris, E. M. J., Shawyer, F., & Farhall, J. (2013). Acceptance and commitment therapy for voices. In E. M. J. Morris., L. C. Johns., & J. E. Oliver (Eds.), *Acceptance and commitment therapy and mindfulness for psychosis* (pp. 95–111). Chichester, UK: Wiley-Blackwell.

Thomas, N., Shawyer, F., Castle, D., Copolov, D., Hayes, S., & Farhall, J. (2014). A randomised controlled trial of acceptance and commitment therapy (ACT) for psychosis: Study protocol. *BMC Psychiatry, 14*, DOI:10.1186/1471-244X-14-198.

van der Gaag, M. (2006). A neuropsychiatric model of biological and psychological processes in the remission of delusions and auditory hallucinations. *Schizophrenia Bulletin, 32*, S113–S122.

van der Gaag, M., Valmaggia, L. R., & Smit, F. (2014). The effects of individually tailored formulation-based cognitive behavioural therapy in auditory hallucinations and delusions: A meta-analysis. *Schizophrenia Research, 156*, 30–37.

Waller, H., Freeman, D., Jolley, S., Dunn, G., & Garety, P. (2011). Targeting reasoning biases in delusions: A pilot study of the Maudsley Review Training Programme for individuals with persistent, high conviction delusions. *Journal of Behavior Therapy and Experimental Psychiatry, 42*, 414–421.

Waller, H., Garety, P. A., Jolley, S., Fornells-Ambrojo, M., Kuipers, E., Onwumere, J., et al. (2013). Low intensity cognitive behavioural therapy for psychosis: A pilot study. *Journal of Behavior Therapy and Experimental Psychiatry, 44*, 98–104.

Walser, R. D., & Pistorello, J. (2004). ACT in group format. In S. C. Hayes & K. D. Strosahl (Eds.), *A practical guide to acceptance and commitment therapy* (pp. 347–372). New York: Springer.

Walsh, J., & Boyle, J. (2009). Improving acute psychiatric hospital services according to inpatient experiences: A user-led piece of research as a means to empowerment. *Issues in Mental Health Nursing, 30*, 31–38.

Westrup, D. (2014). *Advanced acceptance and commitment therapy: The experienced practitioner's guide to optimizing delivery*. Oakland, CA: New Harbinger Publications.

White, R. G. (2015). Treating depression in psychosis: Self-compassion as a valued life direction. In B. A. Guadiano (Ed.), *Incorporating acceptance and mindfulness into the treatment of psychosis: Current trends and future directions* (pp. 81–107). Oxford: Oxford University Press.

White, R. G., Gumley, A. I., McTaggart, J., Rattrie, L., McConville, D., Cleare, S., et al. (2011). A feasibility study of acceptance and commitment therapy for emotional dysfunction following psychosis. *Behaviour Research and Therapy, 49*, 901–907.

Williams, J., Leamy, M., Pesola, F., Bird, V., Le Boutillier, C., & Slade, M. (2015). Psychometric evaluation of the Questionnaire about the Process of Recovery (QPR). *British Journal of Psychiatry, 207,* 551–555.

Williams, J., Vaughan, F., Huws, J., & Hastings, R. (2014). Brain injury spousal caregivers' experiences of an acceptance and commitment therapy (ACT) group. *Social Care and Neurodisability, 5,* 29–40.

Williams, K. E., Ciarrochi, J., & Heaven, P. C. (2012). Inflexible parents, inflexible kids: A 6-year longitudinal study of parenting style and the development of psychological flexibility in adolescents. *Journal of Youth and Adolescence, 41,* 1053–1066.

World Health Organization. (1993). *The ICD-10 classification of mental and behavioural disorders: Clinical descriptions and diagnostic guidelines.* Geneva: World Health Organization.

Wykes, T., Hayward, P., Thomas, N., Green, N., Surguladze, S., Fannon, D., et al. (2005). What are the effects of group cognitive behaviour therapy for voices? A randomised control trial. *Schizophrenia Research, 77,* 201–210.

Zettle, R. D., Rains, J. C., & Hayes, S. C. (2011). Processes of change in acceptance and commitment therapy and cognitive therapy for depression: A mediational reanalysis of Zettle and Rains (1989). *Behavior Modification, 35,* 265–283.

Emma K. O'Donoghue, DClinPsy, is a senior clinical psychologist working in community psychosis settings in a South London National Health Service Trust. She has a long-standing interest in using acceptance and commitment therapy (ACT) approaches with clients experiencing first episode and established psychosis, as well as those with bipolar affective disorder. She has coordinated two randomized controlled trials of ACT workshops for clients and caregivers in community psychosis settings, and clients experiencing bipolar. She is also involved in working with service users to facilitate ACT interventions. Emma regularly trains psychologists in ACT for psychosis interventions, and teaches masters and doctoral courses in ACT approaches.

Eric M. J. Morris, PhD, is clinical psychologist and director of the La Trobe University Psychology Clinic in Melbourne, Australia. Eric previously worked as the psychology lead for early intervention for psychosis at the South London and Maudsley NHS Foundation Trust. He has twenty years' experience treating people with psychosis, and their families, using psychological therapies. Eric completed a PhD at King's College London, researching ACT as an individual- and group-based intervention for people recovering from psychosis, and as workplace resilience training for mental health workers. Eric is coeditor of *Acceptance and Commitment Therapy and Mindfulness for Psychosis*, and coauthor of the self-help guide, *ACTivate Your Life*.

Joseph E. Oliver, PhD, is a consultant clinical psychologist and joint director of the Cognitive Behavioural Therapy for Psychosis Post Graduate Diploma program at University College London. He also works within a North London National Health Service Trust, developing training and delivering interventions for people with psychosis. He is director for Contextual Consulting, a London-based consultancy offering ACT-focused training, supervision, and psychological therapy. Joseph is an Association for Contextual Behavioral Science (ACBS) peer-reviewed ACT trainer, and regularly delivers ACT teaching and training in the UK and internationally. Along with Eric and Louise, he is coeditor of the book, *Acceptance and Commitment Therapy and Mindfulness for Psychosis* and coauthor of the self-help book, *ACTivate Your Life*.

Louise C. Johns, DPhil, is a consultant clinical psychologist and British Association for Behavioural and Cognitive Psychotherapies (BABCP)-accredited cognitive behavioral therapist. She works in the Oxford Early Intervention in Psychosis Service, overseeing the delivery and evaluation of psychological interventions for clients and their caregivers, including the training and supervision of staff. She is also an honorary senior research fellow in the department of psychiatry at the University of Oxford, and an associate member of the Oxford Cognitive Therapy Centre. She led on the first UK-funded study to evaluate ACT for psychosis in group settings, and is coeditor of the book, *Acceptance and Commitment Therapy and Mindfulness for Psychosis*.

Foreword writer **Steven C. Hayes, PhD**, is Nevada Foundation Professor in the department of psychology at the University of Nevada, Reno. An author of forty-one books and more than 575 scientific articles, he has shown in his research how language and thought leads to human suffering. He is codeveloper of ACT, a powerful therapy method that is useful in a wide variety of areas.

Index

A

about this book, 2–3
acceptance: ACT process of, 13, 24; approaches based on, 18–20; definition of, 13; radical, 23
Acceptance and Action Questionnaire–2 (AAQ-2), 114
acceptance and commitment therapy (ACT): central processes in, 13; CHIME recovery framework and, 15–16; empirical studies supporting, 11–12; explanatory overview of, 11; mindfulness used within, 14–15; psychological flexibility model in, 12–14; psychosis interventions based on, ix–x, 2, 20–26
acceptance-based CBT (A-CBT), 22
acknowledgments, 221–222
ACT for depression after psychosis (ACTdp), 22
ACT for Life study, 28–30
ACT for psychosis (ACTp), 20–21; ACT processes in, 24–26; adapting ACT for, 23–26; evidence base for, 21–23; group interventions for, 26–31; rationale for using, 16–20; style of therapy in, 26; therapeutic relationship in, 23–24
ACT for Recovery study, 30–31, 41–44; feedback from caregivers, 41–44; outcomes on caregiver well-being, 41; peer support cofacilitators in, 69, 71, 72, 76
ACT for recovery workshops: acute inpatient settings for, 51–65; booster sessions in, 30, 121, 201–220; caregiver support through, 30, 38–49; evaluation of, 109–115; guidance for facilitators of, 95–97; in-session suggestions for, 120–121; overview of protocol for, 119–120; peer-support cofacilitators in, 67–77; phone calls between sessions of, 121; preworkshop orientation to, 120; reviewing with participants, 219–220; supervising facilitators of, 99–109; taster session in, 123–131; training facilitators of, 79–97. *See also specific sessions*
ACT for recovery workshops for acute inpatient settings, 51–65; adaptations required for, 54–62; cofacilitator feedback on, 64–65; content of sessions in, 59–62; format for offering, 57–58; involving ward staff in, 58–59; outcomes from conducting, 62–63; promoting to patients and ward teams, 55–56; reasons for offering, 53–54
ACT for recovery workshops for caregivers, 30, 38–49; composition of, 39; confidentiality issues in, 45; content of, 44–45; development of, 38; follow-up groups for, 48–49; nature of caring relationship considered in, 48; practical issues related to, 49; recruitment for, 38–39; reservoir metaphor used in, 39–40,

125, 136, 224; results of study on, 41–44; time in caregiver role considered for, 47–48; values identification in, 45–47; video on caregiving used in, 47

ACT groups for people with psychosis (G-ACTp), 2, 26–31; development of, 27–31; rationale for using, 26–27

ACT-consistent facilitator behaviors, 107–108

ACT-inconsistent facilitator behaviors, 108–109

active avoidance, 18

active processes, 14; adapting for psychosis, 25–26; definitions for, 13; exercises related to, 195, 209, 216. *See also* committed action; values

activity levels measure, 113

ACTs of ACT Fidelity Measure, 104–109; ACT-consistent facilitator behaviors, 107–108; ACT-inconsistent facilitator behaviors, 108–109; rating scale, 105–107, 253–255

acute inpatient settings, 51–65; adapting ACT for, 54–62; feedback from staff in, 64–65; format of ACT workshops in, 57–58; nature and characteristics of, 51–53; outcomes of ACT workshops in, 62–63; promoting ACT to patients and staff in, 55–56; reasons for utilizing ACT in, 53–54; session content for ACT workshops in, 59–62; staff involvement in ACT workshops in, 58–59

ADAPT study, 22

adherence, intervention, 104

AESOP-10 study, 9

antipsychotic medications, ix, 7

assessments: fidelity, 109; workshop, 110–114, 250–252. *See also* evaluating ACT workshops

audio recordings of sessions, 109

auditory hallucinations. *See* hearing voices

automatic pilot consideration, 128–129

Avery, Natasha, 119

avoidance. *See* experiential avoidance

aware processes, 14; adapting for psychosis, 25; definitions for, 13; exercises related to, 194, 208, 216; skills development worksheet, 261. *See also* mindfulness; noticing

awareness: nonjudgmental, 20; present-moment, 13, 14

B

believability, 23

Bentall, Richard, 83

between-session phone calls, 121

body, mindfulness of, 129–131, 138–139, 203–205, 225–226

booster sessions, 30, 121, 201–220

booster session 1, 201–210; bringing to a close, 210; committed action exercise, 209–210; main purpose and overview, 201; noticing exercise, 203–205; passengers on the bus metaphor, 205–206; review of committed actions, 206–207; skills refresher, 208–209; timeline and materials, 201–202; values exercise, 207; welcome and introduction, 202–203

booster session 2, 211–220; bringing to a close, 220; group role-play, 217–219; main purpose and overview, 211; noticing exercise, 213–214; passengers on the bus metaphor, 217–219; review of committed actions, 215; skills refresher, 215–216; timeline and materials, 211–212; welcome and introduction, 212–213; workshop review, 219–220 breathing exercises: mindfulness of breath and body, 129–131, 138–139, 203–205, 225–226; three-minute breathing space, 166–167, 182–183, 241

Bremner, Georgina, 51

C

caregivers, 33–49; ACT for recovery workshops for, 30, 38–49; challenges experienced by, 34; confidentiality issues of, 45; content of workshops for, 44–45; evidence base on ACT for, 36; follow-up groups for, 48–49; importance of support by, 34; informal, 33–34; length of time spent as, 47–48; nature of caring relationship for, 48; offering separate workshops for, 39; practicalities of workshops for, 49; psychologically inflexible responses of, 36–37; recruiting for workshops, 38–39; reservoir metaphor for, 39–40, 125, 136, 224; responding to needs of, 35; results from ACT for Recovery study on, 41–44; values identification for, 45–47; video on challenges of, 47

CHIME recovery framework, 15–16

Client Satisfaction Questionnaire (form), 250–252

Client Satisfaction Questionnaire–8 (CSQ-8), 114

Clinical Outcomes in Routine Evaluation–10 (CORE-10), 63, 111

Clinical Outcomes in Routine Evaluation–Outcome Measure (CORE-OM), 111

closed workshops, 57

clouds in the sky exercise, 198–199, 213–214, 249

cofacilitators: peer-support, 67–77, 83–84; psychiatric staff, 64–65

cognitive behavioral therapy (CBT), 7

cognitive behavioral therapy for psychosis (CBTp), 9–10; insight cultivated in, 19; therapeutic relationship in, 23

cognitive fusion: caregiver experience of, 37; measure for assessing, 114

Cognitive Fusion Questionnaire (CFQ), 114

committed action: ACTp adaptations related to, 26; booster sessions and, 209–210; dealing with noncompletion of, 97; definition of, 13; facilitator training about, 94–95; of participants in inpatient workshops, 61; reviewing from previous session, 155–157, 176, 192, 206–207, 215; setting for following week, 145–146, 167–168, 184; worksheet for indicating, 260. *See also* values

compass metaphor, 45–46, 94

competence, intervention, 104

confidentiality issues, 45

conflicts, values, 46–47

connectedness, 15

content-based responses, 108–109

D

Deegan, Pat, 67

defusion: ACT process of, 13, 14, 24; definition of, 13; facilitator training and, 93–94; mistaken views about, 93

deinstitutionalization, 52

delusional thinking, 18

developing aware skills worksheet, 261

dialectical behavior therapy (DBT), 15

disengagement, 20

"do nothing" response, 18–19

downloadable resources, 3, 223

driving license worksheets, 197, 262–263

drop-in sessions, 48–49

E

early intervention service, 80
eating, mindful, 152–154, 230–231
emotion, expressed, 35
empowerment, 16
engagement responses, 17–18
evaluating ACT workshops, 109–115; assessment considerations for, 110–111; outcome measures for, 111–113; participant feedback for, 114–115, 250–252; process measures for, 113–114; reasons for, 110
exercise prompt sheets, 223–255; acting out the passengers on the bus exercise, 238–240; ACTs of ACT Fidelity Measure, 253–255; Client Satisfaction Questionnaire, 250–252; clouds in the sky exercise, 249; George's story transcript, 234–235; key messages cards, 246–248; leaves on the stream exercise, 242–243; mindful eating exercise, 230–231; mindful stretch exercise, 228–229; mindful walking exercise, 244–245; mindfulness of breath and body exercise, 225–226; passengers on the bus metaphor, 227; Paul's story transcript, 232–233; pushing against the folder exercise, 236–237; reservoir metaphor, 224; three-minute breathing space exercise, 241. *See also* worksheets
experiential avoidance: caregivers and, 37; passive vs. active, 18
experiential learning, 24
experts by experience. *See* peer-support cofacilitators
expressed emotion, 35

F

facilitators of ACT workshops: general guidance for, 95–97; mental health professionals as, 82–83; peer-support cofacilitators as, 67–77; self-disclosure by, 24, 120–121; supervision of, 99–109; training of, 79–97
Family and Friends Test, 114
family interventions, 10, 35
feedback: caregiver, 41–44; cofacilitator, 64–65, 73–75; participant, 114–115, 250–252; popcorn, 131, 147, 169, 185, 210
fidelity: ACTs of ACT Fidelity Measure, 104–109, 253–255; helping facilitators run workshops with, 103–104; opportunities to assess, 109
fight responses, 17
fight/struggle scenario, 164–165, 181, 218, 238–239
flight responses, 17
focus in workshops, 95–96
follow-up groups for caregivers, 48–49
fusion. *See* cognitive fusion

G

G-ACTp. *See* ACT groups for people with psychosis
George's story transcript, 234–235
giving-in scenario, 165, 181, 218, 239
goals: driving license worksheet on, 197, 262; setting SMART, 145; values distinguished from, 45–46, 96
ground rules for sessions, 135
group interventions: ACT for psychosis recovery using, 2, 26–31; acute inpatient settings for, 51–65; caregiver workshops as, 38–49; CBT for psychosis using, 7; creating the environment for, 96; peer-support cofacilitators in, 67–77; supervising facilitators of, 99–109; training facilitators of, 79–97. *See also* ACT for recovery workshops
group processes, 43–44

group role-play, 163–167, 179–182, 217–219, 238–240

H
having vs. buying thoughts exercise, 178–179
Hayes, Steven C., xi, 68
health problems, 8
hearing voices, 17–18, 19; acceptance of, 19; responding to, 17–18
Hearing Voices Network, 67
hope, maintaining, 16

I
identity, positive, 16
informal caregivers, 33–34
inpatient settings. *See* acute inpatient settings
inquiry, mindful, 87–89
insight, cultivation of, 19
interviews, cofacilitator, 70
Intervoice: The International Hearing Voices Network, 19

J
Jolley, Suzanne, 33

K
key messages cards, 194–195, 246–248

L
learning by addition, 24
leaves on the stream exercise, 174–175, 242–243
Lifengage trial, 22
Longden, Eleanor, 67

M
Mad Pride movement, 67
Madness Explained (Bentall), 83
Manchester Short Assessment of Quality of Life (MANSA), 112–113
May, Rufus, 67
meaning, finding, 16
measures: outcome, 111–113; process, 113–114
mediation analyses, 22–23
medical model of care, 82
medications, antipsychotic, ix, 7
mental health professionals: therapeutic relationship with, 23–24; training as workshop facilitators, 82–83
mental well-being: ACT for caregivers and, 36, 41; caregiving challenges and, 34; outcome measures of, 111–112; psychological flexibility and, 1, 10
metaphors: compass, 45–46, 94; reservoir, 39–40, 125, 136, 224; two mountains, 23–24, 69. *See also* passengers on the bus metaphor
mindful inquiry: leading exercises on, 87–89; self-disclosure and, 89
mindfulness, 14–15; adapting in ACT for psychosis, 25; caregiver reflections on, 42; developing aware skills worksheet on, 261; facilitator practice of, 89–90; introducing in taster session, 129–131; leading exercises on, 86–89; measure for assessing, 63, 113–114; values-based behavior and, 92–93. *See also* noticing
mindfulness exercises: mindful eating, 152–154, 230–231; mindful stretch, 143–145, 228–229; mindful walking, 190–192, 244–245; mindfulness of breath and body, 129–131, 138–139, 203–205, 225–226. *See also* noticing exercises
mindfulness-based cognitive therapy (MBCT), 15
mindfulness-based interventions (MBIs), 20

mindfulness-based stress reduction (MBSR), 15
mistimed responses, 108
Morris, Eric, 80
mortality, psychosis and, 8

N

National Registry of Evidence-based Programs and Practices (NREPP), x
nonjudgmental awareness, 20
noticing: encouraging self-practice of, 90–91; introducing the concept of, 86, 128–129, 136–137; linking values-based actions to, 92. See also mindfulness
noticing exercises, 25; caregiver practice of, 42; clouds in the sky, 198–199, 213–214, 249; key points for leading, 86–87; leaves on the stream, 174–175, 242–243; mindful eating, 152–154, 230–231; mindful stretch, 143–145, 228–229; mindful walking, 190–192, 244–245; mindfulness of breath and body, 129–131, 138–139, 203–205, 225–226; noticing others' values, 193; three-minute breathing space, 166–167, 182–183, 241

O

observing workshop sessions, 109
Oliver, Joseph, 80
open processes, 13–14; adapting for psychosis, 24; definitions for, 13; exercises related to, 194, 208, 216. See also acceptance; defusion
openness response, 165–166, 182, 219, 239–240
outcome measures, 111–113; of activity levels, 113; of engagement in personal recovery, 113; of interference from symptoms and problems, 112; of quality of life, 112–113; of well-being, 111–112
outcomes of ACT workshops: for acute inpatient settings, 62–63; for caregivers, 41; measures for assessing, 111–113

P

parent caregivers, 36
participants: feedback on satisfaction of, 114–115, 250–252; promoting workshops to eligible, 55–56; reviewing workshops with, 219–220
passengers on the bus metaphor: caregiver feedback on, 43; centrality of, 91; defusion related to, 93–94; description of, 29; exercise prompt sheet for, 227; fight/struggle scenario, 164–165, 181, 218, 238–239; giving-in scenario, 165, 181, 218, 239; group role-play exercise, 163–167, 179–182, 217–219, 238–240; introducing in sessions, 127–128, 141–142; openness scenario, 165–166, 182, 219, 239–240; reviewing key elements of, 154–155, 196, 205–206; video on, 58, 128, 142, 157–160; worksheet on, 259
passive avoidance, 18
passive engagement, 18
patients: promoting ACT workshops to, 55–56. See also participants
Paul's story transcript, 232–233
peer-support cofacilitators, 67–77; background to the role of, 67–68; discussing expertise of, 102–103; feedback on use of, 73–75; lack of professional knowledge/training, 102; need for flexibility with, 72–73; payment offered to, 71; personal accounts from, 74, 75–76; reasons for using, 68–69; selection of, 70–71;

supervision of, 72, 101–103; training of, 71, 83–84
person-based cognitive therapy (PBCT), 20
phone calls, between-session, 121
popcorn feedback, 131, 147, 169, 185, 210
present-moment awareness, 13, 14
preworkshop orientation, 120
problem-solving stance, 96
process measures, 113–114
production line mentality, 52
prompt sheets. *See* exercise prompt sheets
psychiatric inpatient settings. *See* acute inpatient settings
psychoeducation interventions, 35
psychological flexibility, 1; ACT hexaflex model of, 12–14; caregiver responses and, 36–37; mental well-being and, 1, 10
psychological interventions, 9–10
psychosis: acceptance approaches for, 18–20; ACT approach to, ix–x, 2, 20–21, 26–31; early intervention service for, 80; mindfulness-based interventions for, 20; outcomes following, 8–9; prevalence and costs of, 8; psychological interventions for, 9–10; symptoms of, 8, 112
psychosis recovery: definitions of, 9; promoting practice oriented to, 81–82; study on rates of, 9
pushing against the folder exercise, 160–163, 236–237

Q

quality-of-life measure, 112–113
Questionnaire About the Process of Recovery (QPR), 113

R

radical acceptance, 23
randomized controlled trials (RCTs), 21–23. *See also* research studies
recording workshop sessions, 109
recovery: promoting practice oriented to, 81–82. *See also* psychosis recovery
recovery workshops. *See* ACT for recovery workshops
rehospitalization rates, x, 21–22
relational frame theory (RFT), 11
research studies: on ACT for caregivers, 36; on ACT for psychosis, 21–23; on efficacy of ACT interventions, 11–12; on G-ACTp interventions, 28–31
reservoir metaphor, 39–40, 125, 136, 224
resistance strategies, 17
resources, downloadable, 3, 223
role-play exercise, 163–167, 179–182, 217–219, 238–240

S

safe space, 103
safety-seeking behaviors, 17
scaffolding, 26, 91
self-as-context, 13, 14
self-disclosure: facilitator, 24, 120–121; mindful inquiry and, 89
sessions: booster, 30, 121, 201–220; drop-in, 48–49; ground rules for, 135; observing, 109; phone calls between, 121; recording, 109; taster, 30, 123–131
session 1, 133–147; automatic pilot consideration, 136–137; bringing to a close, 146–147; committed action exercise, 145–146; ground rules discussion, 135; main purpose and overview, 133; mindful stretch exercise, 143–145; mindfulness of breath and body exercise, 138–139;

noticing exercises, 137–139, 143–145; passengers on the bus metaphor, 141–142; reservoir metaphor, 136; timeline and materials, 133–134; values consideration, 139–141; warm-up exercise, 135–136; welcome and introduction, 134

session 2, 149–169; bringing to a close, 168–169; committed action exercise, 167–168; group role-play, 163–167; main purpose and overview, 149; mindful eating exercise, 152–154; noticing exercises, 152–154, 166–167; passengers on the bus metaphor, 154–155, 157–160, 163–167; review of committed actions, 155–157; three-minute breathing space exercise, 166–167; timeline and materials, 150; video vignette, 157–160; welcome and introduction, 151–152; willingness exercise, 160–163

session 3, 171–185; bringing to a close, 185; committed action exercise, 184; group role-play, 179–182; having vs. buying thoughts exercise, 178–179; main purpose and overview, 171; noticing exercises, 173–175, 182–183; passengers on the bus metaphor, 179–182; review of committed actions, 176; sticky labels exercise, 177–178; three-minute breathing space exercise, 182–183; timeline and materials, 172; welcome and introduction, 173

session 4, 187–200; bringing to a close, 200; clouds in the sky exercise, 198–199; driving license worksheet, 197; key messages exercise, 194–195; main purpose and overview, 187; mindful walking exercise, 190–192; noticing exercises, 189–192, 193, 198–199; passengers on the bus metaphor, 196; reflection on workshop learning, 197; review of committed actions, 192–193; timeline and materials, 188; values and actions exercise, 193; welcome and introduction, 189; workshop summary, 199–200

session worksheets. *See* worksheets
severe mental illness, 8
Sheehan Disability Scale (SDS), 112
skills refresher, 208–209, 215–216
SMART goals, 145
social recovery, 9
Southampton Mindfulness Questionnaire (SMQ), 63, 113–114
sticky labels exercise, 177–178
stretching, mindful, 143–145, 228–229
stuckness, 69
suicide risk, 8
supervising workshop facilitators, 99–109; ACTs of ACT Fidelity Measure for, 104–109, 253–255; fidelity considerations in, 103–104; group meetings for, 100–101; peer supporters and, 72, 101–103; safe space provided for, 103
symptoms of psychosis, 8, 112

T

targeted interventions, 10
taster session, 30, 123–131; automatic pilot consideration, 128–129; bringing to a close, 131; intended purpose, 123; mindfulness exercise, 129–131; passengers on the bus metaphor, 127–128; reservoir metaphor, 125; timeline and materials, 123; values consideration, 125–127; welcome and introduction, 124
Taylor, Rumina, 51
telephone calls, between-session, 121

therapeutic relationship, 23–24
therapeutic style, 26
therapists. *See* mental health professionals
thoughts: delusional thinking and, 18; exercise on having vs. buying, 178–179
three-minute breathing space exercise, 166–167, 182–183, 241
Time Budget Measure, 113
training workshop facilitators, 79–97; defusion exercises for, 93–94; experiences of authors with, 80–81; general guidance to offer in, 95–97; goals of sessions for, 84–85; ideas on barriers and values for, 91; introduction process for, 85; mental health professionals and, 82–83; mindfulness and noticing exercises for, 86–91, 92; peer supporters and, 71, 83–84; values and committed action for, 92–93, 94–95
transitional discharge, 56
treatment of resistant command hallucinations (TORCH), 22
two mountains metaphor, 23–24, 69

U

Understanding Psychosis and Schizophrenia (British Psychological Society), 83

V

values: ACTp adaptations related to, 25–26; barriers to, 126, 140–141; caregiver connection with, 37, 42–43, 45–47; conflicts between, 46–47; definition of, 13; driving license worksheet on, 197, 262; exercise on exploring, 207; facilitator training about, 94–95; goals distinguished from, 45–46, 96; identifying in ACT, 14; introducing the concept of, 125–126, 139–140; noticing others' actions and, 193; of participants in inpatient workshops, 60; worksheet for identifying, 140, 258
values-based actions: linking noticing and willingness to, 92–93; measure for assessing, 114; SMART goals for, 145. *See also* committed action
Valuing Questionnaire (VQ), 63, 114
video recordings of sessions, 109
videos: on caregiving challenges, 47; on passengers on the bus metaphor, 58, 128, 142, 157–160
voices. *See* hearing voices

W

ward staff: involving in ACT workshops, 58–59; promoting ACT workshops to, 55
Wardwick-Edinburgh Mental Well-Being Scale (WEMWBS), 111
warm-up exercise, 135–136
web resources, 3, 223
well-being. *See* mental well-being
willingness: linking values-based actions to, 92; pushing against the folder exercise, 160–163, 236–237
workability, ACT emphasis on, 20
worksheets, 257–263; committed action, 260; developing aware skills, 261; driving license, 197, 262–263; passengers on the bus, 259; values, 140, 258. *See also* exercise prompt sheets
workshops. *See* ACT for recovery workshops

MORE BOOKS from
NEW HARBINGER PUBLICATIONS

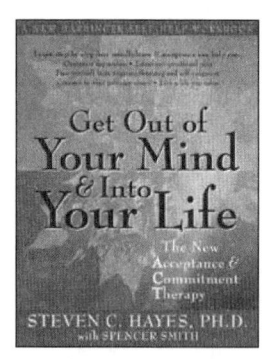

GET OUT OF YOUR MIND & INTO YOUR LIFE
The New Acceptance & Commitment Therapy
978-1572244252 / 21.95

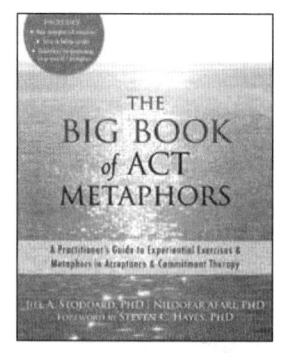

THE BIG BOOK OF ACT METAPHORS
A Practitioner's Guide to Experiential Exercises & Metaphors in Acceptance & Commitment Therapy
978-1608825295 / US $49.95

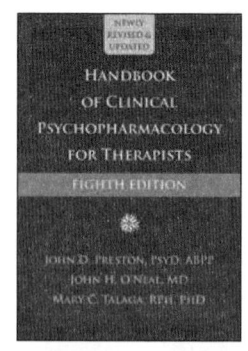

HANDBOOK OF CLINICAL PSYCHOPHARMACOLOGY FOR THERAPISTS, EIGHTH EDITION
978-1626259256 / US $59.95

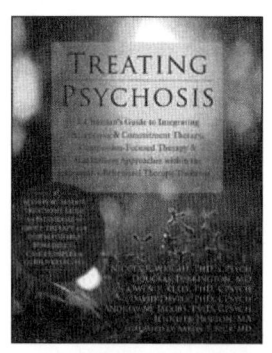

TREATING PSYCHOSIS
A Clinician's Guide to Integrating Acceptance & Commitment Therapy, Compassion-Focused Therapy & Mindfulness Approaches within the Cognitive Behavioral Therapy Tradition
978-1608824076 / US $49.95

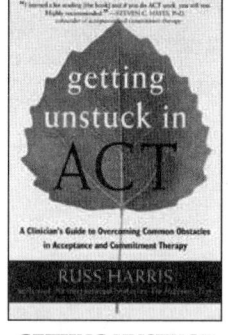

GETTING UNSTUCK IN ACT
A Clinician's Guide to Overcoming Common Obstacles in Acceptance & Commitment Therapy
978-1608828050 / US $29.95

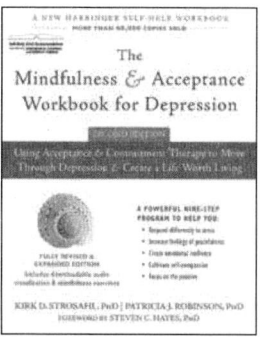

THE MINDFULNESS & ACCEPTANCE WORKBOOK FOR DEPRESSION, SECOND EDITION
Using Acceptance & Commitment Therapy to Move Through Depression & Create a Life Worth Living
978-1626258457 / US $24.95

newharbingerpublications
1-800-748-6273 / newharbinger.com

Follow Us

(VISA, MC, AMEX / prices subject to change without notice)

Sign up to receive **Quick Tips for Therapists**—
fast and free solutions to common client situations mental health professionals encounter. Written by New Harbinger authors, some of the most prominent names in psychology today, Quick Tips for Therapists are short, helpful emails that will help enhance your client sessions.

Sign up online at **newharbinger.com/quicktips**

Sign up for our Book Alerts at **newharbinger.com/bookalerts**